RWANDA

History and Hope

Margee M. Ensign and William E. Bertrand

University Press of America,® Inc.
Lanham · Boulder · New York · Toronto · Plymouth, UK

Copyright © 2010 by
University Press of America,® Inc.
4501 Forbes Boulevard
Suite 200
Lanham, Maryland 20706
UPA Acquisitions Department (301) 459-3366

Estover Road
Plymouth PL6 7PY
United Kingdom

Library of Congress Control Number: 20099636356
ISBN: 978-0-7618-4942-1 (clothbound : alk. paper)
ISBN: 978-0-7618-4943-8 (paperback : alk. paper)
eISBN: 978-0-7618-4944-5

⊖™ The paper used in this publication meets the minimum
requirements of American National Standard for Information
Sciences—Permanence of Paper for Printed Library Materials,
ANSI Z39.48-1992

Dedication

To all those who are rebuilding Rwanda

Contents

Tables and Figures

Foreword

BY PAUL KAGAME,
PRESIDENT OF THE REPUBLIC OF RWANDA

This work constitutes an important contribution to debate, discussion and policymaking in our country through its thorough analysis of socioeconomic and political developments and challenges in Rwanda in the recent past. The authors are correct in saying, "We are accustomed to hearing and accepting negative news, particularly when it refers to Africa." Few realize that the continent has experienced significant and positive changes in a process that began to gather momentum with the defeat of the apartheid system in South Africa in 1994 and the rise of a society and leadership committed to reconciliation and democracy—an experience that became widespread in much of Sub-Saharan Africa in the 1990s.

That very same year of the end of apartheid, Rwanda was engulfed by a genocide whose sole purpose was to eliminate all Tutsi. We were left to fight alone as the world looked silently on.

But from the ashes we have made significant progress in building a unified and reconciled nation as the authors analyze and describe—our efforts have centered on rebuilding our socioeconomic fabric, and in creating stronger national institutions to take our nation forward with greatly improved capabilities to improve lives of Rwandan people.

Our experience in the last fifteen years demonstrates that a landlocked nation—rising out of a crisis—through the use of informed strategy and timely action, can grow. And that through growth, we can eradicate poverty, and create a society that shares power, is more broadminded and accepting in terms of differences, and more trusting, action-oriented, and self-determined.

We realize in Rwanda that the challenges ahead will require even more determined efforts to create prosperity to lift our people out of poverty. Professors Ensign and Bertrand arrive at the same conclusion with our vision 2020—they rightly point out that productive sectors, in particular efforts to modernize our agriculture, are critical next steps to increasing incomes of the poor, since that is the sector from which most of Rwanda's population earns its living.

This book, like Rwanda's recent history, is one of hope. The Rwandan people have committed themselves to building a society based on peace, justice and inclusiveness because our liberation was not just an armed struggle or an exercise to simply remove bad governments. It was also about ensuring the improved quality of life in our otherwise impoverished nation. In Rwanda we realize that our primary assets reside in our people, and secondarily, in our material resources. Because of our history we have tried to break away from a business-as-usual approach to our development and develop a new path, a new paradigm.

This book goes beyond discussion of symptoms and looks closely at root causes of Rwanda's underdevelopment, and the pathway to a better future. To undertake this important task, the authors invested much time and effort. Their work blends the human stories of reconciliation and rebuilding with what they call "an evidence-based analysis" of Rwanda's progress and continuing challenges.

Rwandans and those who follow developments in our country should find this work invaluable—it should not only set standards in academia, but also provide powerful tools for improving informed policymaking in our country through its insights and ideas.

Acknowledgments

The authors are very grateful to their colleagues in Rwanda, the United States, and Europe who contributed to this book including: Bonaventure Niyibizi, Maggie and Christine Baingana, Romain Murenzi, Rose Kibuye, Davinah Milenge, Daphrose Gahakwe, Protais Musoni, Jeanne d'Arc Mujawamariya, Ambassador David Macrae, the students at FAWE, Professors Cort Smith, Mathilde Mukantabana, Jean-Pierre Karegeye, and Dr. Eamon Kelly at Tulane University. Dorothy Albritton provided outstanding assistance as our editor. Dr. Ensign would also like to thank the faculty and staff at the School of International Studies at the University of the Pacific and Provost Phil Glbertson for their support and understanding, Dr. Julie Sina at UCLA, her parents and family for their inspiration, and daughter, Katherine for her commitment to social change and development.

Introduction

Bonaventure

"I didn't do my homework," the student said. "But Bonaventure," I replied, "You can't get behind in this course." "I need to go home. I think my family is going to be killed."

That conversation, close to fifteen years ago, changed my life. Bonaventure Niyibizi was a senior Foreign Service National (FSN) in a course funded by USAID, and taught by a group of development experts in Washington D.C. The Development Studies Program (DSP) brought together senior employees working for the US government overseas, especially those in poorer countries, for an intense, seven-week course. The faculty came from numerous disciplines: economics, political science, sociology and health. We were the "experts" talking about economic, political and social development in these countries. Like so much in academia, the true experts were the students. The conversation with Bonaventure was one of those "aha" moments when I realized how little I really knew about the countries that formed the bases of our lectures.

I drove Bonaventure to Washington Dulles airport with another student, Henderson Patrick[1] and we put him on a plane to Kigali. The rest is history. But is it? While the world turned a blind eye—except for the French who actively supported the genocidal Hutu government—Bonaventure and thousands of Rwandans tried to survive unimaginable violence. Many who survived are part of the greatest experiment in reconciliation and rebuilding the world has witnessed.

I tried to forget what might have happened to Bonaventure and went on with my life and career. But I could not forget his comments, his smile, and his determination. My co-author encouraged me to uncover what had happened to him. So in 1999, six years after putting Bonaventure on a plane, I decided to go to Arusha, the site of the United National International Criminal Tribunal for Rwanda (ICTR), to try and comprehend the incomprehensible that had occurred during those three horrific months in 1994, when an estimated one million Tutsi's and moderate Hutu's were hacked to death.

I sat for days and listened as the most barbaric stories emerged—how brothers killed each other and their parents; how young girls and women were gang raped, and how women helped to organize the genocide.[2] Once again, the world was absent. Often I was the only spectator going back and forth between the different courtrooms. As Samantha Power noted in "Rwanda: The Two Faces of Justice," "But, as with the genocide itself, the world has shown little interest in the criminals who carried it out. More than five hundred journalists descended on The Hague to cover the start of the Milosevic trial in February 2002; just forty came to Arusha to cover the launch of the trial of Bagosora, a man few outside Rwanda would be able to identify as the genocide's leading culprit."[3]

On the fourth day of my visit to the ICTR, a young man approached me. "Why are you here? He asked. "Few from the West have visited these trials." I told him my story about Bonaventure and that I assumed he had died. "He is alive!" the man exclaimed, "and he is the Minister of Commerce in President Bizimungu's Cabinet." That day I flew to Kigali, the capital of Rwanda. I was checking into the Hotel Mille Colline, the basis for the story Hotel Rwanda, when I heard a voice behind me, "What are you doing here, Dr. Ensign," I turned and saw Bonaventure. "I came here to find you, "I said between tears. We hugged, cried, and later that day went for coffee.

He told me his story: what had happened when he returned from the course, how the situation deteriorated and the killings escalated up to April 1994. He recounted what happened when the Embassy evacuated all of the Americans and left behind all the Rwandan employees. He shared his 100 days of terror and how he came back and started working again—for USAID—in July 1994, in the same building where thirty of his colleagues had died. He explained how he and his family survived. First they hid in their house. Eventually they took in twenty friends and neighbors. At the height of the killings, as a last hope, Bonaventure went to seek assistance from a UN captain who lived in his neighborhood to try to reach the Mille Colline hotel. A Hutu neighbor[4] intervened and told the UN official they were all Tutsi. The UN captain asked Bonaventure if he was Tutsi. "I said yes. He asked me if all twenty I was hiding were Tutsi. I said yes. He asked if we had changed our ID cards. I said no." 'Then I can't take you. We will take only Hutus, Zairois and Burundians and no Tutsi. I could leave a UN flag at your house!'" Bonaventure went back to his house in despair. The following day another Hutu neighbor came. "You are the only one remaining on the list in the neighborhood—you have no chance to survive," he said.

"That was one of the lowest days of my life," said Bonaventure. But he devised a plan with his friends to reach the Sainte Famille Church. "We were sure that our chances were tiny, but we chose to be provocative and die by bullets instead of by machetes." They got into three cars and divided the families so at least one member of each family might make it. They drove quickly. The first two cars made it. "Mine was stopped at a roadblock, down the hill from the Mille Colline. The killers were singing the extermination songs aimed at sensitizing the population to kill all the Tutsi's. They had machetes and grenades and they were drunk. A military convoy with armored vehicles came by and distracted them. We made a quick run to the church. We made it, but many people, men and women, were lying dead on the roadside. This was just a few days after the beginning of the genocide."

The Sainte Famille Church is a short distance from the Mille Colline Hotel, where Tutsis were seeking refuge, but it might well have been a continent away. There were roadblocks and killers outside the Church. Bonaventure and his family blended in with the 2000 or so taking refuge in the Church. On April 15th in the morning, he was outside, hiding with his sons, when he decided to bring them back inside the small chapel. Sainte Famille was suddenly invaded by militias, policeman and presidential guards. They started selecting the Tutsis and brought them outside where they were killed and their bodies put in a mass grave nearby. Bonaventure had barely made it inside. He was on their list of people who had to be killed that day. Toward the end of the day he saw one of the Interhamwe (which means those who attack together in Kinyarwanda) militiamen walk by the window with a list of names. His name was first on the list. "A Hutu who had sought refuge because he was married to a Tutsi told the militia that I had been taken by the presidential guard. The militia put a line through my name. We were saved for that day and we had to move that night for another place to hide. I found out later that my mother was not saved; she was killed on April 16th."

He told me what happened when the Americans came back to Rwanda. "They were prepared to grant me and my family asylum in the United States," he said. "Why didn't you take it? How could you stay here," I asked. His simple answer is the story of post-genocide Rwanda: "Who would rebuild this country if we all left. Our fellow Tutsi who had left in the 60s and 70s were coming back. There were a lot of orphans and widows. I needed to stay to help rebuild Rwanda," he said forcefully.

I knew that day that we needed to hear Bonaventure's story, and the many more who survived and are rebuilding their lives and their country. I have had the opportunity to travel and work in Rwanda for more than a decade and marvel each visit at how far and fast the country has progressed.

In December 2006, on a month long visit to Rwanda, I called Bonaventure, He sounded very tired and anxious. I knew he had just started a new job as President of a bank in Kigali. He was also trying to finish an MBA. He told me that this was not the source of his anxiety; that his mother's killers had been identified and that their Gacaca trial had begun. The second hearing was the following week. It was difficult for his family to attend the hearing, he said, and to hear the testimony. I asked if it would help if I went with him. "Yes," he said.

We traveled two hours from Kigali, inland, on steep roads to the site of Bonaventure's mother's home. Just outside the village we stopped to wait for two filmmakers Bonaventure had hired to film the proceedings. We talked about a new referendum that was being discussed that would ban the death penalty in Rwanda. I asked him how, as a victim, he felt about banning the death penalty. "I have never been for the death penalty but we must fix prison sentences so that the killers stay and have to think about what they did. We should not be pressured by the UN and humanitarian groups to release them."

When we arrived in the village, a hush went through the large crowd that had assembled for several trials that day. Gacaca, which means grass in the local Kinyarwanda language, is Rwanda's attempt to deal with over a million people charged with murder, rape and destruction of property during the genocide.

The judges were elected from the village. The government spent twelve years methodically assembling and documenting the cases. Many in the West have criticized this approach because the accused have no lawyers. What alternative does this poor country have to find some form of justice and to offer solace to those who survived when over a million people have been identified as having participated in the genocide?

For six hours in a hot sun, I sat next to Bonaventure as he heard (and translated for me) the testimony. One man was accused of murdering dozens of children by throwing them in the river where they drowned. Another, the bourgomaster or mayor, was accused of finding the Tutsi, including Bonaventure's mother where she was in hiding in a small house with her five grandchildren, and directing the killing.

A pivotal moment came when the bourgomaster said to Bonaventure, "I did not kill your mother but I did kill your nephews' five children." Bonaventure's nephew sat next to us on the small bench.

Eight people were on trial that day for the murders. As we waited for the verdicts, we walked to see where his mother had hid. I saw the small house and could only weep at what had happened there. After conferring for over an hour the seven judges returned to the open area where the trials had occurred—just as the hot sun was setting. The crowd was silent. Babies were hushed, and all stood to hear the verdicts.

These eight people were their neighbors, their friends, their husbands, brothers and sisters. And those who were killed had been their neighbors all their lives, generation after generation. Until that moment, all of those waiting for the verdict had spent the last year living freely in the village. This is why what is unfolding in Rwanda is unprecedented.

After World War II, the post-genocide countries of Europe had few survivors to integrate into their societies. This is not the case in present-day Rwanda where the perpetrators of genocide are facing the survivors in these community-based trials. Many of the perpetrators have already been released into their communities—serving part of their sentences as community service. No society has ever attempted what this poor country is now facing—reconstructing individual lives and rebuilding an economy and political structures while including many of those who participated in the genocide.

We stood as the chief judge; a young, serious woman announced the verdicts.

All were guilty but only two had to serve more time. The others had also committed indescribable crimes but they had confessed according to the Gacaca law. The two men who had to serve more time in prison had not confessed and they were sentenced to thirty additional years in prison. (The Gacaca law was later revised and those who appealed were sentenced to less than twenty years—although nothing had changed in their being convicted of killing) The two men who were found guilty were sentenced to thirty additional years in prison.

At the end of the day, we followed the truck, over steep roads, as the two convicted murders were taken to the local prison, a small wooden structure not far from the village. Bonaventure wanted to make sure they were put immediately behind bars.

"I feel free now," he said. "I know who killed my mother and now I feel free."

On the way home we visited a new house that he is building in his village. "My family has had to rebuild it six times since 1960," he said. "Six times they have torn it down and in the end they exterminated my family here." "Who are they I asked." "They are the villagers who are angry at me for testifying." "Aren't you afraid? Why are you rebuilding?" "That would mean giving in to them," he replied.

Next to his new house is a church. "My mom gave the brother of one of the people who came to kill her a cow because his children had been dying of starvation. When we were sitting in the church right after the genocide, their father confessed to me that his children were among those who killed my mother. On his way to kill my mom he stopped at this church."

Bonaventure's life story is the story of Rwanda. The actions of the Catholic Church, the French, the Americans, and his life as a refugee and now bank President, are all part of the mosaic that contributes to Rwanda's history and its current status.

When he was six years old, in 1959, he hid in the bush for the first time. A priest, Father DuChamp, came to his village with a crowd of killers. His role was to shoot in the air to threaten those in hiding. "We were afraid to death and left the bush. They told all the men to come forward. The crowd of killers murdered many of them. Those who tried to escape were hunted down and thrown in the Nyabarongo River. More than thirty years later, the same scenario was repeated; this time they left no one to survive. "Few in the world are aware of the role that many priests and nuns played before and during the genocide.[5] We all need to ask ourselves how *Thou Shall Not Kill*, became, *You Will Kill*.

Like many Tutsi's, Bonaventure and his family left Rwanda during the early 1960s. Eventually, he and his family came back to their village in the mid-1960s and he pursued his primary school and then went to the seminary. In 1972, all Tutsi who had scored high on the tests were expelled from the seminary by the priests. "Father Vianney Rusingizandekwe and Archbishop Andre Perraudin, a Swiss, did this to us. There was no place to go. I could not enroll in school; I could not get a job." In despair he left Rwanda and went to Zaire, where he pursued his studies. He returned in the early 80s. "I could not find a job, the segregation was in place." Finally he found a small job working for USAID. He quickly rose through the ranks. In the early 1990s he was imprisoned for being too close to the Americas, for being disloyal. When he got out in 1992, his house was attacked mid-day by government soldiers seeking to eliminate him. He was not there but his son was left with grenades. In 1993, he was sent to the US to take the Development Studies classes. I did not realize when he was a student in Washington DC that winter that he had just been released from six months in prison.

The remnants of a colonial, French speaking administration, the destructive power of the French and the Church, retribution, revenge and reconciliation, all of this is the history of Rwanda.

None of us can imagine what Bonaventure and many others lived through, and what they continue to experience every day. The horror for many is unspeakable. What we can do is to give survivors and those who died a voice. We can document how Bonaventure and others are rebuilding their lives and their country, to bring to life the tremendous hope that exists, and progress that is occurring, in this small, landlocked country in Central Africa.

A few years after the genocide, Bonaventure was in Nairobi on business. He walked by someone begging on the street. "It was the person from my neighborhood who had betrayed me and my family when I was seeking assistance from the UN captain. He looked so hungry; I gave him some money for food." This is forgiveness.

Much remains to be done. Rwanda is still very poor. Gacaca has been controversial; some of the witnesses have been killed. Bonaventure has been threatened again. Yet, as Bonaventure said, "who else is going to do this work?"

In November 2008, Bonaventure stood on his patio in his backyard overlooking Kigali. The city lights were sparkling. A group of twenty people, American investors, an Indian-American banker and Rwandan friends laughed and chattered about building a movie theatre in Kigali. "I never thought I would see the city like this again. There is so much progress and change," Bonaventure said. This is hope.

Notes

1. Henderson Patrick went on to become the Mission Director for Rwanda after the genocide. He and Bonaventure have remained very good friends.

2. See Landesman, Peter "The Minister of Rape." *New York Times Magazine*, September 15, 2002, 82-89.

3. Samantha Power, "Rwanda: The Two Faces of Justice." *The New York Review* (January 16, 2003): 47.

4. See the end of this introduction. Bonaventure met this same Hutu neighbor a numbers of years later in Nairobi.

5. See Carol Rittner, John K. Roth and Wendy Whitworth, *Genocide in Rwanda: Complicity of the Churches?* Newark, U.K.: Aegis Publishers, 2004.

Chapter One

Acknowledging Progress and Emphasizing Evidence

Imagine a nation with the highest proportion of women legislators in the world. Imagine a country where a democratically elected president is committed to gender equality and poverty reduction, where urban and rural schools are being wired to the Internet, and where the government is committed to becoming a knowledge-based economy and middle income country by 2020. Imagine that this country is located in the heart of sub-Saharan Africa and that this progress comes in the wake of one of the 20th century's worst nightmares.

Fifteen years removed from a mass genocide that resulted in the deaths of nearly one million people, Rwanda today presents a model for hope, justice, innovation and human development. In fact, Rwanda is now a leader in achieving economic, political and social progress in this beleaguered continent. A new model of governance has emerged in this poor, African country. This model, that draws on century's old Rwandan customs called Ubudehe and Imihigo, is inclusive, transparent, empowers the poor and holds leaders accountable for improving the well being of people in their districts. No other country has developed and implemented such an innovative development program.

Going around the United States talking to various groups, we have discovered that these paragraphs may be difficult for many in the West to accept. We are accustomed to hearing and accepting negative news, particularly when it refers to Africa, the second largest continent in the world composed of 54 different states. The terms *failed state, AIDS pandemic*, and *war* and *conflict* are among the most frequently used terms and concepts when discussing this large continent, especially in the Western media. When one of the authors made a presentation on progress in Rwanda to a group of foundation employees charged with funding projects on the continent, she was told simply that the story couldn't possibly be true-this was Africa, this was Rwanda. Potential editors said more than once, this book contradicts everything we have heard about Rwanda.

Africa is the second largest continent in the world. All of the United States, Europe, India, China and Argentina would fit comfortably in this large landmass. Yet, most of what people in the West are exposed to in the media reflects only the problems and tragedies: AIDS, famines, and corruption. The stories frequently come from what American stars are doing in Africa: from Madonna in Malawi to George Clooney in Darfur and Angelina Jolie meeting with refugees as the goodwill Ambassador for the UN High Commissioner for Refugees. These stars usually present a continent in need of "saving," a place full of tragedies and turmoil. As one blog on global refugees stated:

> Angelina Jolie is a caring individual who's willing to take the time to promote public awareness of a good cause—even if it means putting herself in undesirable and sometimes risky conditions.

Newsweek's story about the star was titled, "Angelina Jolie Wants to Save the World."[1]

Using stars to sell the issues, focusing on individual solutions rather than a larger context, and focusing on dramatic, crisis driven stories has serious consequences for international policy and for individual citizens' efforts to understand real issues. The negative and entertainment-based coverage of Africa by much of the Western press is only the most glaring example of the limited and biased international news currently broadcast.

In 2006 as the US bombed targets in Somalia, Anderson Cooper, one of CNN's anchors said: "We all saw the movie Black Hawk Down and know the consequences of US intervention in Africa." When did movies and entertainment television become the basis for our international knowledge? Entertainment-based or "soft" news media, including shows such as Entertainment Tonight, watched by an estimated 4 million Americans, have grown significantly in the past few decades. What has been called the "Oprah effect" has a significant impact on shaping public opinion towards foreign policy, at least in the US. This type of coverage, often dramatic in nature, usually lacks the larger political, economic and international context. Researchers have found that viewers are often attentive but left without an understanding of the cause and consequences of the stories they are viewing.[2]

Much of the movie Hotel Rwanda was fabricated.[3] Yet many viewers believed the movie was real, and that forms the basis for their knowledge of Rwanda. Religious leaders were portrayed as protecting Tutsis when in reality many religious leaders participated in the genocide, and a number have been convicted of crimes against humanity. The hotel manger was portrayed as a savior when he is accused of extorting money for protection, and one lone UN Ghanaian soldier posted outside the Hotel Mille Colline offered a symbol of protection that kept the killers outside. The real stories would force us to examine and acknowledge the depth of the United States' and the international community's failure in Rwanda.

Africa is not a cause; it is a continent full of smart and dedicated citizens trying to improve their lives and their countries. Africa does not need to be saved by well meaning Westerners whether they are rock stars like Bono or religious leaders like Rick Warren who has declared Rwanda to be his first "Purpose Driven Nation." While Orpah's new school for girls in South Africa offers hope to those attending, it also contributes to a global perception that solutions for Africa will have to come from the West. Because of this stereotype, we miss important, positive stories about progress on the continent that emerge from the people themselves.[4]

Why did few newspapers cover the World Bank announcement in 2007 reporting the positive and very significant news that primary enrollment on the continent has increased sharply in the past decade? Most development experts acknowledge that increasing primary enrollment, especially for girls, is one of the most important investments a developing country can make. Educating girls reduces fertility, infant mortality and malnutrition, and allows half of the population to participate knowledgeably in society. "Primary enrollment rates continent-wide increased from 72 percent in 1990 to 93 percent in 2004. Africa is on the rebound. . . . Africa is today a continent on the move, making tangible progress on delivering better health, education, growth, trade and poverty-reduction outcomes,"[5] noted the World Bank's Report for Africa in 2007. Did you read this story—probably not? Few newspapers reported it.

The Africa Progress Panel, an organization focused on progress and challenges on the continent that is chaired by former Secretary-General Kofi Annan and former British Prime-Minister Tony Blair, said in its 2009 annual report:

> Africa's story remains one of unsteady but remarkable progress punc-
> tuated by setbacks and chronic problems. On the one hand, the conti-
> nent has never been in a better position than today. Not only are there
> more democratic countries than ever before (almost thirty as opposed
> to merely five at the end of the Cold War) and fewer civil wars (three
> as opposed to thirteen a decade and a half ago), but over the past
> decade most countries have also been able to record real progress,
> whether in terms of economic growth and private sector development,
> primary education, women's rights or the fight against poverty and
> disease.[6]

By only covering bad news, we create a continuing climate of despair which has many consequences: brain drain, a savior attitude as
represented by many donor organizations as well as the Hollywood stars
who are depicted as "saving" African orphans, less desire to visit and
enjoy the enormous educational and tourism destinations of the continent, and perhaps most importantly an overall sense of defeatism regarding much needed foreign investment and even humanitarian assistance in
the region.

It is true that most Africans are poor, have less access to health care
and education than most other regions of the world, and many live in
countries where ethnic politics dominate. In the second largest continent
in the world, with over 53 countries and 250 million people, there are
many serious problems. But we have become conditioned to hearing
only the negative stories about African countries and societies, and in
some respects have come to expect them. Worse still, in some cases, as
the authors have discovered first hand, this conditioning has made it
impossible even for people who should know better to take seriously any
positive reports.

The negative bias is even evident in the Millennium Development
Goals (MDGs), a set of targets for reducing poverty by 2015, which
were agreed to at a summit in 2000 convened by the United Nations and
attended by the leaders of 189 countries. By 2005, the MDG reports
were already emphasizing that Africa would not meet any of the goals:

> Africa is the only continent not on track to meet any of the goals of the
> Millennium Declaration by 2015.
>
> (UN World Summit Declaration, 2005)

In Africa . . . The world is furthest behind in progress to fulfill the
MDGs. . . . Africa is well behind target on reaching all of the goals.
(Blair Commission for Africa, 2005)

Sub-Saharan Africa, most dramatically, has been in a downward spiral
of AIDS, resurgent malaria, falling food output per person, deteriorating shelter conditions, and environmental degradation, so that most
countries in the region are on a trajectory to miss most or all of the
Goals. . . . The region is off track to meet every Millennium Development Goal.

(UN Millennium Project,
Investment in Development, Main Report 2005)

As Easterly points out in a thoughtful critique of the measurement
choices of the MDGs, "Many of the choices made had the effect of
making Africa's progress look worse than is justified compared to other
regions. . . . The statement that 'Africa will miss all of the MDGs' thus
paints an unfairly bleak portrait of Africa."[7]

The Millennium Development goal setting exercise in itself[8] has been
an important positive step for the international development community.
The MDGs established a metric that effectively focused the world community on the need to bring the poorest countries and people quickly up
to a minimally acceptable standard of living. Rwanda has invested significant time and resources into incorporating MDG goals into national
reporting. As we demonstrate in this book, contrary to received wisdom
Rwanda is on track to meet many of the Millennium Development Goals,
and should be a case study of the functional integration and implementation of Millennium Development Goals at the national level.

In trying to understand the current state of African countries' political, economic and social development, we often forget the historical
context. Africa was the last region to break the bondage of colonialism.
It was not until the end of World War II that most African countries
achieved independence, at the same time that the US and Soviet Union
faced off around the world. Many African countries became pawns in
the Cold War's division of the world, and social and economic development took second place to issues related to national security policies of
Western countries.

Africa's boundaries were drawn arbitrarily at the Berlin conference
of 1884-85 when Great Britain, France, Belgium, Italy, Portugal, Germany and Spain redrew the boundaries of a thousand indigenous cultures

and superimposed a new map that supported the economic desires of the imperial powers. Colonial powers were interested in extracting resource, not building local capacity in schools, infrastructure and public institutions. Often colonial leaders treated their "subjects" as subhuman.[9] But colonialism ended fifty years ago you might be saying. We would do well to remember where the US and other so called industrialized countries was a short fifty years after independence. In fact, the real end of colonialism was the end of the Cold War, when the Berlin wall crumbled in 1990.

To understand the genocide in Rwanda, we will need to revisit its colonial past. You have almost certainly not heard the true story—and you won't get it by going to your local movie theater. We need to revisit this tragic story to show just how far Rwanda has come in such a short time, and how truly astonishing its progress has been.

The colonial legacy in Rwanda had a profound influence on the evolution of the country and its decent into genocide. Racial prejudice based on ethnic identity was a deliberate strategy used by the colonial powers, by the genocidal Hutu government of Juvenal Habyarimana and by the Catholic Church to legitimize their rule that hardened into hate and revenge in the 1990s. The Church was closely aligned with the Hutus and several priests and nuns have been implicated in assisting the perpetrators, several are awaiting trial, and one Catholic priest was found guilt of crimes against humanity in December 2006.[10] Much of this history, especially the role of the Church, has yet to be written.[11] Yet this deliberate policy, which originated with the Belgian colonial authorities working in conjunction with Church leaders, laid the foundation for the genocide that began on April 7, 1994.

During one hundred days of terror that followed, close to one million Tutsi's and moderate Hutus were slaughtered in Rwanda at a rate greater than the Nazi killing during the Holocaust.[12] It is difficult to overestimate what happened in Rwanda and even more difficult to understand how and why it happened.[13] Scholars from around the world continue to discuss and debate the historical origins and consequences of the genocide. This much is clear—the state sponsored Hutu government set out to kill as many Tutsi's as possible. They succeeded in killing close to a million. The motivations of the state, the Catholic Church, the role of the French and individual participants are extremely complex and are still being unraveled.

The international community, led by the Clinton administration in the U.S., also has significant responsibility for the tragedy.[14] It was very clear in the months leading up to April 1994 that widespread violence was probable. In 1994, with clear knowledge of what was unfolding, the international community turned a blind eye, withdrew United Nations troops and allowed a genocide—organized by the state—to overtake the country. The United Nations had established an independent International Commission in January 1993 to examine the growing violence in Rwanda and had concluded that a "climate of terror" existed in Rwanda and that the government was doing nothing to stop it.

When the genocide erupted, the United Nations, at the insistence of the United States and led by then President William Clinton and Secretary of State Madeline Albright, not only blocked the deployment of additional UN forces that could have protected citizens but lobbied to withdraw all UN troops. "We have to learn when to say no," said President Clinton. The UN's Chief of Peacekeeping at the time, Kofi Annan, ceded to US demands. There is strong evidence that France provided direct military assistance to the genocidal government that continued during the genocide. The UN responded to the crisis by reducing its commitment and allowing the million to be murdered.

Much still needs to be written about how and why this genocide occurred. But this is not that book. It begins as the genocide ended, when visionary leaders stopped, what seemed to outsiders as unstoppable, and asked themselves how Rwanda could be reborn.

That is why this story is an important one. Rwanda is still one of the poorest countries in the world with the majority of its people (90%) dependent on subsistence agriculture. It is a country dealing with the perpetrators of genocide who are now facing their survivors in community based trials. Called Gacaca (Ga-cha-cha), and based on a traditional method of dealing with minor offenses, these community based trials are attempting to met out justice to the perpetrators of the genocide and bring some sense of reconciliation to the survivors.

Many of the perpetrators are being released into their communities—serving part of their sentences as community service. After World War II, the post-genocide countries in Europe had few survivors to integrate into their societies. This is not the case in present day Rwanda that is rebuilding an economy, physical and political structures, while including many of the murderers. No society has ever attempted what this poor country is attempting.

Yet it is a country with a vision and a plan to reach that vision. It is a country full of honest, dedicated leaders who understand that the stakes are high. It is a government that has decentralized power and instituted a way of measuring whether leaders perform as the people expect. Rwandans call this process Ubudehe and the contract that people sign with their leaders, Imihigo.[15] It is a novel method for understanding what poor people want in their lives and ensuring to some degree that leaders respond to their needs. This is worth repeating. Rwanda is implementing a system that asks poor people to express their needs that are then developed into a compact—called Imihigo—with their leaders—who are held accountable, by being removed from office by citizens if these needs are not met. This is not just a theory: we have watched it in action. In 2008, the Ubudehe program was awarded the United Nations Public Service Award. 150 countries participated in the program, 12 were nominated and Ubudehe took first place.[16]

According to the United Nations:

> The prize recognises global excellence in public service in countries around the world. "Ubudehe" programme empowers citizens at community level in Rwanda to plan and implement poverty reduction projects. The programme was found to have fostered citizens' participation in policymaking while having improved transparency, accountability and responsiveness in the public service. . . .

Commenting on this award, European Commissioner for Development and Humanitarian Aid, Louis Michel, said:

> This innovative programme empowers people at the grassroots-level to play an active role in tackling poverty head-on. This trophy is a major recognition of the essential role local communities play in development. The EU strongly supports this kind of people-focused approach to create the right conditions for development.

For Sub-Saharan Africa and for all poor developing countries Rwanda is demonstrating a new model of development: a model that is unique and innovative in several respects.[17] It is a country that has built a vision and a strategic plan with the active involvement of its poor citizens. It is a vision and a plan that recognizes the key roles of information technology, education, health, and gender equity in reducing poverty and improving lives.[18] A country of a little over 9 million people, it is dealing with justice for thousands involved in the genocide and reconciliation for the survivors. It is a vision that includes indigenous elements as well as drawing on the successful experiences of other countries that have moved from poor to prosperous.

Rwanda is a story of how a governing philosophy has emerged that harkens back to the thinking and writings of Aristotle and Rousseau; how an economy is being rebuilt based on the 21st century digital revolution and a social contract focused on human development. It is a story of how the basic necessities of life: an educational system based on tolerance, widespread access to primary health care, and explicit policies to create an equal society for men and women, is unfolding and still being written.

Rwanda is a story about accountability. At every level of government, leaders are being held accountable for their goals, objectives and performance. A feedback and accountability mechanism is built into leaders' performance contracts. Data for monitoring and evaluation for all major government projects are gathered by the National Bureau of Statistics and then transmitted to leaders from the grassroots to the Parliament and the President.[19]

Rwanda's commitment to building a world-class, nation-wide statistical system was recognized by the World Bank in 2007. Every year the World Bank ranks all countries in the world on several dimensions of statistical capacity. Rwanda along with Nigeria showed the biggest improvement in performance moving from 23 in Africa in 2006 to 6 in 2007.[20] There is not other developing country in the world that uses monitoring, evaluation, and accountability in this way.

Ubudehe and Imihigo, results-based performance for governance,[21] are not only making a difference but are replicable in every country of the world. Finally it is a story of committed, visionary, educated leaders, many who grew up outside of Rwanda, but who fought to stop the genocide and stayed to rebuild the country.

But this is not a story without evidence. It is not a case story of how one person made a difference building a network of schools or providing money for medicines. There are numerous inspiring stories of how individuals make a difference in the lives of the poor; in fact they dominate much of the popular literature on global poverty. But there is a large and growing disconnect between the evidence of what works on a large scale to improve the lives of poor people and individual stories of good intentions.

This gap in understanding can be attributed, in part to the rise in "soft," dramatic news but also to the failure of academics, like us, to make the knowledge and evidence that has developed over the past five decades widely available to interested individuals and groups. Sometimes our vocabulary and our writing styles prevent otherwise interested and well-intentioned parties from understanding the evidence of what works. And there is a large body of research and evidence that should guide policy and projects, development assistance and evaluation. This book is an attempt to tell an evidence-based story of Rwanda in a way that is accessible not only to academics but also to interested students of development.

The overwhelming evidence from countries and regions where poverty has been reduced and life expectancy increased in the last decades, from China to Vietnam points to the essential role of the state in ensuring that access to education and health care is widespread, that girls and women benefit equally, and that economic growth is pro-poor. The history of developing pro-poor economic and social policies which included universal access to education and health care emerged after World War II in countries that were devastated by that war. The so-called Asian tigers, using strong and capable bureaucracies, developed a deliberate set of programs and policies that focused on mobilizing savings and investment, and integrating these growing economies with the international trading system while expanding access to education and health. Because the population was increasingly educated and healthy, when economic growth took off, the benefits were widely shared. South Korea, Taiwan, Singapore, Hong Kong (the original Four Tigers) and now China, Malaysia, Indonesia and increasingly Vietnam and Thailand, are on their way to becoming middle-income countries.[22]

Many of these countries, such as Korea and Taiwan, in their initial phase of development were authoritarian. China, where poverty reduction efforts, especially in rural areas, have been stunning (dropping from 250 million in 1978 to approximately 26.4 million in 2001), remains deeply authoritarian. Are there poverty-reduction lessons for Africa from China?[23]

Many, especially those in the human rights community, have accused Rwanda, and President Kagame of being authoritarian, of running a one-party state. But they have not looked at the evidence. Many in this community have allowed themselves to embrace the conventional wisdom that arose soon after the genocide ended. Based on the extensive evidence outlined in this book, that conventional wisdom is simply wrong.

Certainly Rwanda has taken a very hard, principled stand on how it thinks it should deal with the perpetrators, and the "culture of impunity" that led in part to the genocide, and has been resistant to calls from the West to follow a traditional model of justice and reconciliation. The Director of the Irish Centre for Human Rights and the National University of Ireland, in an article discussing post-genocide justice in Rwanda says:

> Everybody talks about battling impunity, but few societies have done this with greater determination or more stubborn resistance to compromise than Rwanda. . . . Rwanda's approach to transitional justice is one of the most principled manifestations of the commitment of international human rights law and policy. While many other post-conflict societies have delayed, postponed and even prevaricated, resisting the admonitions of various international organizations, personalities and NGOs, Rwanda has insisted upon holding perpetrators accountable.[24]

Tom Ndahiro, a survivor, a former member of the Human Rights Commission in Rwanda, author, and someone who was interviewed extensively for this book, wrote a recent article about those who are reinterpreting the genocide and post-genocide period in Rwanda. Comparing them to money launderers, he says:

> The list of those who have laundered the 1994 genocide of Tutsi is long. Many of these individuals and organizations have gained great credence in the international community. As early as April 1994, various state governments and the United Nations were comfortable sitting with the orchestrators of the genocide . . . and many . . . have become prominent genocide launderers. The UNSC (Security Council) listened to their interpretations of the violence occurring in Rwanda and invited them to negotiate peace agreements. The international media, particularly French news agencies, aided the denial of the genocide as it was unfolding, by characterizing the violence as simply the spontaneous of ancient, tribal hatred. . . . The UN endorsed the French government's humanitarian mission, Operation Turquoise, thought its impact was decidedly inhuman, creating a security cordon through which tens of thousands of Hutu, including many orchestrators of the genocide, fled to Zaire, (now the Democratic Republic of the Congo). . . . The responsibility for countering the spread of hate propaganda

and new waves of genocidal ideology fell to the living victims and the Rwandan Patriotic Front (RPF), which had defeated the genocidal armed forces and halted the murder of Tutsi and their sympathizers. As the world focused on the plight of Hutu refugees in the camps in Zaire and Tanzania, and unwittingly helped feed, clothe and re-arm them through humanitarian aid, the RPF and genocide survivors were left to rebuild Rwanda and to safeguard it against the re-emergence of genocide ideology.[25]

Support for the "genocide launderers" interpretation of the genocide and post-genocide developments in Rwanda is strong. One of the reasons we have taken close to a decade to complete this book is because of the desire to ensure that the analysis and conclusions are supportable and backed by strong evidence. The work has been painstaking and thorough. Rwanda is being rebuilt by the survivors, by the refugees who have returned home and with the support of many international donors. Besides building a system for dealing with the perpetrators (Gacaca) they have rebuilt the justice sector and drawing on some of the elements of the East Asian development model, especially the emphasis on education, health care and the role of information and communication technologies (ICT) have crafted a new model of governance that is inclusive, transparent and results-oriented.

In fact, if democracy is defined as holding leaders accountable for the wishes of the people, Rwanda, unlike the East Asian countries at an earlier stage of economic and social development, has decentralized power and authority and is developing a new approach to democratic accountability. In fifteen years, the government and people of Rwanda have developed a vision for their country, written a constitution, established free primary education for all children, and have experienced eight years of strong economic growth. The country is laying a foundation for information technology that will result, eventually, in much of the country being connected to the Internet. Women are involved, and in many fields dominate decision-making at the highest levels. This is a country that despite the savagery of the genocide realizes that its people are its primary strength.

Yet enormous challenges remain. Close to 70% of the population lives below the poverty line.[26] Life expectancy is one of the lowest in Sub-Saharan Africa. Thirteen percent of the urban population is infected with HIV/AIDS. Rwanda has one of the highest population growth rates in the world—growing at close to 3% a year—and as a result is doubling its population every 23-25 years. This rapid population growth is one of the most serious challenges and if not controlled could undermine any progress in poverty reduction.

Organized religion, a primary source of violence during the genocide, is resurgent. Fundamentalist groups, coming from Europe, Canada and the U.S. with authoritarian structures and gospels, are active throughout the country. While decentralization has been underway for a decade, and to an extent greater than other poor countries, poor people's voices are being heard, poverty remains a major challenge. The justice sector, while far more independent than at any other time in Rwanda's history, needs far more education and training for its judges. A major consequence of the genocide is that trained professionals, especially in the justice sector, are a scarce resource. Finally, Rwanda, like most poor countries has few natural resources. While the economy has grown, questions remain about the sustainability of that growth. There are serious environmental concerns and while Rwandan coffee is a success story, agriculture is far from producing enough food for the country.

There are many who say that the gains to date are not sustainable, that a society cannot truly reconcile and rebuild after genocide, for people to forgive or live with the killers and build a peaceful and sustainable society. Perhaps we need to listen to the voices of Rwanda as we assess the evidence of their post-genocide success:

"No one reacted," Bonaventure said when the killing began. "No one reacted when we asked for help from the UN. Now we must rebuild our society for our children."

There is much to learn about rebuilding, reconciliation and hope from the people of Rwanda, and much to learn from the evidence-based story of post genocide Rwanda.

Notes

1. See Daniel Drezner, "Foreign Policy Goes Glam," *The National Interest* (2007).

2. Matthew Baum, ""Circling the Wagons: Soft News and Isolationism in American Public Opinion," Paper delivered at the 2002 meeting of the American Political Science Association and Matthew Baum, *Soft News Goes to War:*

Public Opinion and American Foreign Policy in the New Media Age. Princeton: Princeton University Press, 2003.

3. Willis Shalita, "The Fallacy of the Movie Hotel Rwanda." Paper presented at the Post-Genocide Conference, California State University, Sacramento, California November 22-3, 2007. Interviews with survivors who were in the Hotel Mille Colline (the basis for the film) are consistent in their stories of what happened: the hotel manager not only did not help those in the hotel, he extorted money to protect them.

4. See Hunter-Gault, Charlayne. *New News Out of Africa: Uncovering Africa's Renaissance.* New York: Oxford University Press, 2006, and President Ellen Johnson Sirlief in Sirlief, Ellen Johnson and Steven Radelet. "The Good News out of Africa: Democracy, Stability and the Renewal of Growth and Development," in *Visions of Growth: Global Perspectives for Tomorrow's Wellbeing* edited by Beatrice Weder di Mauro Berlin: Campus Verlag, 2008, for introductions to progress in parts of Africa.

5. "World Bank Sees Africa Progress." BBC News, August 7, 2007.

6. Africa Progress Panel: An *Agenda for Progress at a Time for Global Crisis. Annual Report of the Africa Progress Panel*, Geneva, Switzerland, 2009. Also see www.africaprogresspanel.org.

7. Easterly, William. "How the Millennium Development Goals are Unfair to Africa." Brookings Institution Global Economy and Development Working Paper 14. (November 2007).

8. See Ashwani Saith, "From Universal Values to Development Goals: Lost in Translation." *Development and Change* Vol. 37, No. 6 (2006): 1167-1199.

9. See Hochschild, Adam. King Leopold's Ghost: A Story of Greed, Terror and Heroism in Colonial Africa. New York: Houghton Mifflin, 1998 for the story of Belgian colonialism in the Congo.

10. "Catholic Priest Found Guilty in Rwanda Genocide." *Washington Post*, December 14, 2006, P. A20.

11. Tom Ndahiro, one of the country's first human rights commissioners, has been systematically gathering and compiling the history of the genocide, especially the role of the Catholic Church and the French. The one book to date that begins to document the Church's role is Rittner, Carol John K. Roth and Wendy Whitworth. *Genocide in Rwanda: Complicity of the Churches?* Newark, U.K.: Aegis Publishers, 2004. See in particular Fowler, Jerry. The Church and Power: Responses to Genocide and Massive Human Rights Abuses in Comparative Perspective." and Ndahiro, Tom "The Church's Blind Eye to Genocide in Rwanda." In Rittner, Carol John K. Roth and Wendy Whitworth *Genocide in Rwanda: Complicity of the Churches?* Newark, U.K.: Aegis Publishers, 2004.

12. See Gourevitch, 1998.

13. For a comprehensive description of the genocide see Melvern, Linda *Conspiracy to Murder: The Rwandan Genocide.* London: Versco, 2004.

14. See Samantha Power, *"A Problem from Hell": America and the Age of Genocide.* New York: Harper Collins, 2003; Melvern, L.R. *A People Betrayed: The Role of the West in Rwanda's Genocide.* London: Zed Books, 2000; and the National Security Archive www.nsarchive.org that contains thousands of pages of US government records on the Rwandan genocide.

15. Government of Rwanda Vision 2020 Umurenge: An Integrated Local Development Program to Accelerate Poverty Eradication, Rural Growth and Social Protection." EDPRS Flagship Program Document, August 2007, and Ensign, Margee. "Imihigo and Local Governance in Rwanda." Presented at the Urban Institute, Washington D.C., April, 2007, and Carpio, Maria Abigail. "VUP Financial Services Component: Proposed Framework and Operating Guidelines." *Oxford Policy Management,* February 2009.

16. European Commission, Rwanda Program Scoops Top UN Award, AllAfrica, July 2, 2008. See chapter three, pages 79-80 for a more thorough discussion of the UN Award.

17. Fritz, Verena and Alina Rocha Menocal "Developmental States in the New Millennium: Concepts and Challenges for a New Aid Agenda." *Development Policy Review* Vol. 25, No. 5 (2007): 531-552.

18. International Monetary Fund. *Final Evaluation Report of Rwanda's Poverty Reduction Strategy (2002),* July, 2006 for a comprehensive summary of Rwanda's poverty reduction strategy, progress and challenges in reducing poverty.

19. United Nations Economic Commission for Africa: African Centre for Statistics: "Special Focus Africa in Global Statistical System." Volume 2 Issue 1 (March 2008) 1-52.

20. World Bank, (2007) Rwanda Country Economic Memorandum, Washington D.C. World Bank, "Doing Business: Rwanda in Top 20 Reformers Globally," December 3, 2008. http://www.worldbank.org/WBSITE/EXTERNAL/COUNTRIES and "World Bank Sees Africa Progress." BBC News, August 7, 2007.

21. For the best introduction to this new literature on performance-based governance see, Julnes, Patria de Lancer, Frances Stokes Berry, Maria Aristigueta, and Kaifeng Yang eds. *International Handbook of Practice-Based Performance Management* London: Sage, 2008.

22. This is discussed more thoroughly in Chapter two but also see Nanak Kakwani, and Ernesto Pernia. "What is Pro-Poor Growth?" *Asian Development Review* Vol. 18, No. 1 (2000): 1-16; Raphel Kaplinsky and Dirk Messner. "Introduction: The Impact of Asian Drivers on the Developing World." *World Development* Vol. 36, No. 2 (2007): 197-209. Ndulu, Benno *Challenges of African Growth: Opportunities, Constraints and Strategic Directions.* Washington, D.C.: The World Bank, 2007.

23. See Ravallion, Martin. Are There Lessons for Africa from China's Success Against Poverty? World Bank Policy Research Working Paper No. 4463, Washington D.C., The World Bank, January 2008.

24. William A. Schabas, "Post-Genocide Justice in Rwanda: A Spectrum of Options." In Phil Clark and Zachary Kaufman eds. *After Genocide: Transitional Justice, Post-Conflict Reconstruction and Reconciliation in Rwanda and Beyond*. New York: Columbia University Press, 2009.

25. Ndahiro, Tom. Genocide-Laundering: Historical Revisionism, Genocide Denial and the Rassemblement Republicain pour la Democratie au Rwanda." In Clark, Phil and Zachary Kaufman eds. *After Genocide: Transitional Justice, Post-Conflict Reconstruction and Reconciliation in Rwanda and Beyond*. New York: Columbia University Press, 2009, p. 103.

26. International Monetary Fund and International Development Association. *Joint Staff Advisory Note of the Poverty Reduction Strategy Paper: Annual Progress Report*. March 27, 2006.

Chapter Two

A Framework for Assessing Progress in Rwanda

How does one evaluate progress in a country that experienced one of the worst genocides of the twentieth century? What standards are appropriate and where does one begin? As we shall see, there has been very little agreement in the West or elsewhere about what it means to "develop" or what economic, political and social "progress" might be, or how we might measure it. How much more difficult, then, it will be to ask and answer such questions about a country recovering from civil war and genocide.

Can a society that has been torn apart by mass conflict simultaneously deal with justice and reconciliation while building a foundation for equitable and sustainable economic growth? Can programs and policy be developed from the grass roots in a country where brothers and sisters killed each other and their parents? Can gender equity be achieved in a place where women were often the worst of the organizers and the killers?

Rwanda is facing all of these challenges and more, yet it has made much progress. But what do we mean by progress? What values and standards should be used to evaluate "development" in any country in the world, but especially one that had to rebuild almost its entire human and physical infrastructure? Should progress be assessed relative to other countries in the region or at a similar level of economic, political and social development? Is the process of development to be assessed by using the international standards that have evolved during the past six decades of development? Is there agreement on the framework underlying these standards?

For the past six decades the development industry, led primarily by the major funders—the World Bank, the International Monetary Find and in the early decades, the U.S. Agency for International Development (USAID) has scripted the story of growth and development. In the 1950's-60's, state planning and economic growth based on industrialization were the mandated and supported strategies. Most developing countries were viewed in a pre-capitalist state, and with sufficient external resources would be able to generate sufficient economic growth and "take-off."

In the 1970s' when the scope of poverty in poor countries became evident as new data sources emerged, providing for what was called the basic needs of populations in education, food, health care, shelter, and employment became the focus of international donors and policy advisors. This strand of thought, that development progress is primarily about improving the individual quality of life, remains an important goal for developing societies as well as motivation for development assistance.

In the 1980s when the price of oil increased dramatically, and internal and external resources for development dried up, reducing the role of the state and opening economies up to global competition became the policy prescriptions. During this same decade a different model of development, based on state control of economics and politics emerged. Other countries in the region quickly followed the so-called Asian Tigers policies. The Asian model—successfully growing their economies while reducing poverty—offers important lessons for building a framework for evaluating development policies. This same decade saw the beginning of a strong environmental movement that has forced us to ask serious questions about sustainability and the relationship between economic growth and the environment.

The roles of government and politics, especially building democracy, are threads woven throughout the past sixty years of development. Human rights were an important part of President Carter's foreign policy legacy. At the end of the 20th century, notions of governance and human rights combined with an emphasis on accountability and transparency dominated. At the beginning of the 21st century, a focus on human development and decentralized governance and empowerment started to take center stage.

In late 2007, a global economic crisis began to spread like a tsunami across the world. The impact of this crisis is only beginning to be felt in the poor countries. Whether it will fundamentally alter the lessons from sixty years of development thought and practice remains to be seen.

A careful evaluation of each of approaches offers important lessons and evidence for building a framework for evaluating progress in human development. Because, in fact, there are no globally acceptable standards for defining, measuring or evaluating the processes and goals of development. The Millennium Development goals, which were agreed to by the international community in 2000 are the closest we have to judging the goals of development, but even these are not universally accepted, nor do they offer a clear conceptual framework for evaluation. This is not to say that the goals are not important ones, but the list of goals and objectives does not constitute a conceptual or causal framework for understanding why the goals are important, how they affect other goals, and misses key elements that sixty years of research has shown to be important in supporting what we call broad-based and sustainable development. Moreover, none of the millennium standards capture the historical, often colonial legacy that continues to shape the development process, especially in Sub Saharan Africa.

For the last 60 years, people have been struggling with the question of what it means to become "developed" and how we might measure it. First they argued that it was emulation of the Western industrial model, and then the focus and priority shifted to taking care of the most basic needs. The role of the state, how the international economy affects development priorities and possibilities and what is means for people to participate in decisions that shape their lives, have all become part of the development model. But none of the existing models offer a way to understand or explain how a country should proceed in the wake of genocide. Yet this is exactly the challenge that Rwanda's leaders faced in July 1994 when all of the economic, physical and human capital was destroyed.

This chapter examines the evolving model for development and draws out the empirical evidence of what has worked to improve people's lives in poor countries. Based on this evidence, it concludes with a set of five questions that are used to evaluate Rwanda's development performance since the genocide of 1994. In the rest of this chapter we will discuss development theory as it is now understood among professionals in the field. For those less interested in "development theory," feel free to skip to the next chapter where we will focus on the analysis of Rwanda in earnest.

Six Decades of Development

Development thinking, policies and aid strategies have changed radically since the field of development economics emerged at the end of World War II.[1] They have changed based on new ideas and theories, and on evidence that has emerged with the gathering of new data. Sometimes the shifts in thinking and policy are based on the evidence of what works, more infrequently, on lessons learned from failures. Especially during the Cold War, lasting approximately from 1950-1990, ideology, not empirical findings, motivated development assistance and policy of bilateral aid donors and the international financial institutions. Because most developing countries at the time of independence had little trained human and financial capital, development assistance had a significant impact on the direction of domestic programs and policies.

The major exceptions were the East Asian countries—societies that had been devastated by World War II—that followed a path not dictated by the international financial institutions and aid donors. The "success stories" of these countries combined very high rates of economic growth with unsurpassed reduction in poverty and improvements in human well-being. In fact it is notable that the Asian societies have progressed the most during the past six decades, in terms of rapid growth with poverty reduction. Important lessons can be learned from the successes and failures of these countries development strategies.

In the early post-war decades, the field of development studies and policy was dominated by economics. In last few decades, the approach to understanding development has become more multi-disciplinary. In fact the history and evolution of development thinking can be traced from a preoccupation with economics in the first few decades, to a widening that included, over time, perspectives from public health and education in the 1970s, then anthropology, sociology, political science and environmental science in the 1980s and 1990s.

While the field of development studies is far richer than it was in earlier decades because of the entrée of new disciplines, many of the important findings that are now available are often inaccessible to policy makers and interested citizens. Scholars continue to write for people and journals in their own field and practitioners often don't access the research that could make a difference to policy development and analysis. This book is a small attempt to derive the lessons from each relevant area and develop a conceptual framework that can help assess progress in

Rwanda and other countries. The lessons from each decade of development, the evidence of what has worked and what has not in improving human welfare can form the basis of a conceptual framework for evaluating development progress.

1950-1960: Development as Economic Growth and Modernization

In the early post-independent decades of the 1950 and 1960s, growing the economy was equated with development. W. Arthur Lewis' dual model for economic development and titles like *The Industrialization of Backward Areas* reflected the dominant development theory and strategy that was called the modernization paradigm. The path to development involved rapid industrialization and drawing resources from the traditional agricultural sector, which was seen as backward and characterized by low productivity. It was assumed countries would grow if they invested in building roads, bridges and machinery. All that poor countries needed to do to ensure growth in gross national product (GNP) and development was for the state to accumulate capital, invest and industrialize. Since the developing countries, by definition were poor, and could not generate much domestic savings, the gap in what was needed for growth (which was never clearly specified) would be met with external financing provided by foreign aid donors.

To be eligible for foreign assistance, donors required that developing countries develop detailed economic plans for the future that would be implemented by a centralized state, before aid would be dispersed. In 1963, then Secretary-General U Thant stated in the preface of a report entitled, *Planning for Economic Development*:

> the importance of national planning for economic development is almost universally recognized today. . . . Numerous developing countries as well as more advanced economies have employed planning as a tool for achieving their national goals.

Unfortunately, however, the theories and data required for building these models simply did not exist. Nevertheless, the "financing gap" model (also called the Harrod-Domar model) became the primary planning tool for donors and development experts. This simple idea—growth is proportional to investment—held reign for many decades, and was simply wrong.

Sixty years later we know the impact of this strategy: in many of the poor countries and regions, despite billions in assistance to fill the financing gap, poverty has increased. The industrialization strategy, with its single minded approach on state-led capital accumulation, ignored much of what we now know is required for countries to become wealthy and improve the quality of life of their citizens: the political and economic structures of society, the importance of building human capital and ensuring that men and women have equal access to education, health care, and employment; the role that agriculture plays in reducing rural poverty, and the key role of technological change.

Growth is essential for improving a country's standard of living. But generating economic growth is much more complicated than these simple, but influential models, understood and predicted. Growth is essential for poverty reduction but not sufficient. These early models assumed that the benefits of growth would "trickle down" to the poor. Most poor countries belied that assumption. A country's GNP can grow rapidly, without the benefits of that growth being shared widely in the population.

There are obvious examples in the developing world of countries that have performed quite impressively in terms of economic growth, such as Brazil, but have very high poverty and abysmal income distribution figures. On the other hand there are countries such as Costa Rica whose growth rates have not been as strong as others, but who have very impressive records in terms of human and social development. If growth does not lead automatically to improvements in incomes, education, and health, then is not likely to be sustainable in the long run. Moreover inequity in the distribution of income may increase the likelihood of conflict in a society and makes those with less income more vulnerable to natural disasters. Growth is necessary but not sufficient. The type of growth matters. Rwanda's economy has grown quite dramatically in the past seven years. How much have the poor benefited from this economic take-off?

The evidence from this decade also shows the key role that agriculture plays in building food security as well as incomes. Many of the poor in the world live in rural areas and are involved in subsistence farming. Improving farming techniques and productive capacity through new technologies and extension efforts not only lead to increases in production, but also boost incomes and reduce poverty. Because of the negative biases against agriculture and toward industrialization evident in this early period of development, many poor countries entered the 21st century in positions of serious food insecurity with high levels of rural poverty.[2] Rwanda is still primarily a rural society with pockets of deep poverty. What is Rwanda's strategy and success in growing sufficient food and improving the incomes and lives of those in rural areas?

It is in evaluating the success of the Asian economies, that we are coming to understand growth policies that reduce poverty. A pro-poor growth strategy involves adopting policies that build on a country's comparative advantage, which is labor in most poor countries, increasing productivity in agriculture through appropriate inputs and resources, establishing a stable macro economy, and more direct policies such as government spending for basic education, health and family planning, and assuring access to credit. These are the important early lessons about economic growth and development.[3]

During the late 1960s, as more data and information began to emerge, the preoccupation with economic growth began to shift to a focus on equity, poverty basic needs and employment.

1970: Basic Human Needs

Data for understanding the processes of development only began to materialize in the 1970s. Before this time useful data was scarce except for measuring economic growth. Little empirical information was available for leaders and researchers to use for making decisions or analyzing the impact of those decisions. Publication of one of the first wide scale surveys in the developing world surprised many. A 1969 report of the International Labor Organization showed that poverty was widespread in many developing countries and that small numbers were employed in the so called modern sector with the majority of the labor force, which lived in rural areas and worked in agriculture, living in abject poverty.[4] In part because of this new information, new development strategies were adopted and supported by external donor agencies in the 1970s.

During the 1970s, the buzzwords were growth with equity, redistribution with growth, basic human needs and the beginning of a focus on women in development.[5] Improving access to health care and protecting the environment surfaced toward the end of this era. The basic needs strategy that emphasizes literacy, shelter, food and employment for the poor, remains a strong paradigm in development theory and practice.

Only in the early part of the 21st century was this focus on improving the lives of the poor, merged with the necessity of a growing economy (that was pro-poor), good governance and individual rights.

Growing Populations

During this 1960s and 1970s, it also began to be very clear that global population was exploding.[6] In the 1950s, the population of the world numbered about 2.5 billion. As public health programs were increasingly successful in reducing the death rate (with better sanitation, more access to clear water, and the introduction of antibiotics) populations exploded because birth rates did not fall as fast as death rates.

By 2006 the global population had tripled, reaching 6.6 billion people. The majority of the globe's population, 5.4 billion, lives in the developing world. China (at 1.3 billion) and India (1.1 billion) constitute close to 40% of global population and almost a half of the developing countries.

Many of the problems we associate with the poor countries can be laid at the feet of this positive development: improvements in human life that resulted in fewer people dying and more babies living. While most regions of the world have reduced their birth rates, and fertility rates for women are at replacement level fertility in much of the developing world, this is not the case for much of Sub-Saharan Africa, and especially for Rwanda.

A crucial set of policies to achieve sustainable human development then, are population policies. It is obviously easier to achieve higher standards of living if the population is not doubling every generation. Every time the population doubles, a society must provide twice the infrastructure, twice the social services, and twice the production of basic needs, just to keep the standard of living from deteriorating.

Numerous research findings are very clear on how fertility is reduced: female education, combined with access to family planning and reproductive health care are the key interventions required for reducing female fertility.[7]

It is critical then that women have absolute and unrestricted access to the services and information they need to reduce their fertility to whatever level they desire. The most fundamental population policies are legal reforms and health service enhancements that make birth planning information and services available to all women who wish to use them. No less important as population policies are development policies that speed the demographic transition by providing women with education and employment opportunities, so they have other avenues to economic and social advancement. Then the desired, optimal number of children begins to decline.

Because of numerous cross-national research projects that began during this decade we now understand that female education has far more positive consequences. When girls and women are educated, infant and child mortality is reduced. Female education, and more recently an understanding of the importance of gender equity are two of the most important empirical lessons emerging from this decade that have been verified many times by researchers.

Gender Equity

A 1975 United Nations Conference in Mexico was a turning point in development. The conference brought together women from around the world to discuss the status of women. The discovery that in the majority of countries women have fewer rights, work harder and longer hours, at a lower rate the men, led to an entirely new perspective on half of the world's population. The focus shifted from the biological differences between men and women to the gender roles that are constructed by society and culture.

Since the 1970s, we have learned that gender equity matters. Educated women have healthier, smaller and better-educated families. Increasing access to education for girls and women also increases individual, family and national income.

Gender equity provides even more benefits. A study of one hundred countries found that educating girls and improving gender equity promotes democracy. This same World Bank study found that countries that promote women's rights and increase their access to education and economic resources, grow faster, and have less inequality than countries that do not support women's' rights.[8]

Moreover, studies are finding that women may also be the "fairer" sex: having more women in government is associated with lower levels of corruption. More women in government and politics equal more honest government. Countries with fundamentalist regimes—those where terrorism is more likely to be generated—are those where women's participation in social and political life is the most restricted. Working to increase women's voice and participation is far more likely to lead to democracy than forced attempts at voting. In fact if gender inequity if not reduced, sustainable development and democracy may not be possible.

A key component of building a conceptual framework for analyzing development progress in Rwanda, and in any country in the world, is the extent of gender equity.

Healthy People

Good health is an end in itself as well as instrumental in reducing poverty and inequality. Research findings from around the world have documented the impact of improved health outcomes—such as reducing infant and child mortality—have on reducing poverty, fertility, and supporting economic growth. Evidence from East Asia documents that improvements in health, education and gender equity were widespread and supported the economic take off. More specifically, in these high growing economies, as life expectancy increased by one year, GDP increased by 4%. For many years the conventional wisdom was that good health was "affordable" only when countries began growing rapidly.[9] It turns out the opposite is true: healthy people can go to school, learn more, and become productive workers and involved citizens. Late in the 1990s, economist Jeffrey Sachs documented what applied scientists and health professionals had known for decades and that was the importance of basic health as the foundation for development. The development of an indicator called the DALY or disability life adjusted year is now an indicator accepted by all development professionals.[10]

Education

Educated citizens are the foundation of any society. Citizens who have knowledge and skills are better able to evaluate information and make better decisions for their own lives. Higher levels of education transform attitudes, behaviors and expectations and open up economic and social opportunities for people. We know that educating girls and women leads to reductions in fertility, child malnutrition and HIV/AIDS prevalence.

Education is also one of the essential vehicles for development in a society. Higher levels of education are associated with reductions in poverty and improved economic growth.[11] Because of all the positive consequences of education, increasing access to education has been an important objective for the past sixty years. The focus in most developing countries has been ensuring that all children are enrolled in primary school, and is one of the Millennium Development Goals. It is clear, however, that this level of education is far from sufficient for an individual and a country. In the digital age where knowledge has become as important as other factors of production, developing not just literacy, but proficiency in science and technology may be a key determinant of an individuals and a country's success. Has Rwanda invested in science and technology as well as basic education?

The 1970s laid the groundwork for an approach to development that emphasized the importance of education, good health, population reduction and gender equity—all interventions that should lead to poverty reduction. Numerous studies have confirmed that widespread access to education and health care, and gender equity are three key interventions for ensuring broad-based and sustainable development. Rwanda's progress and challenges in these areas form an important part of the framework for evaluation.

The impact of OPEC's price increases, and the debt crisis that was its consequence washed away much of the progress of this decade and led to a new ideology about how countries should "develop."

1980: Macroeconomic Reform, Reducing the Role of the State and the Emergence of Asian Tigers

Few development challenges of the past six decades have had more of an impact on the developing world than the oil price increases of the1980s. OPEC countries first doubled the price of crude oil and then doubled them again in the 1980s. A global recession followed. Many poor countries borrowed from private international banks to try and keep development strategies on track, and in many cases to line the pockets of dictators. Countries that had not been deemed creditworthy before the price hikes suddenly were able to access million of dollars in credit lines. OPEC's banking systems were undeveloped so they recycled their profits with the international private banks, which then were predominately American, who then lent them out in dollars at variable interest rates.

This borrowing became unsustainable as the global economy declined, interest rates soared, and borrowers were unable to export and pay back their dollar denominated loans. The debt situation became a debt crisis when the Mexican foreign minister arrived in Washington in 1982 and announced that his country could no longer pay back their debts to the predominately American banks.

The solution that emerged was for the IMF to purchase this debt in exchange for radical changes in the way developing countries ran their states and their economies. Libraries are full of the analyses of the impact of the debt crisis and the impact of policies developed by the international financial institutions to deal with these structural problems.[12] What became known as the Washington Consensus became the new development paradigm. The policy prescriptions were fixed and one size fits all: reduce the role of the state, reorient public expenditures, liberalize economies and open them to foreign trade and investment, privatize state-owned enterprises, and deregulate.

The overwhelming consensus is that not only did this strategy not work, the list of policy prescriptions led to increased poverty in most of the developing world. The specific political, historical, social and cultural contexts of countries were ignored. Equally important the Washington consensus was not well grounded in the reality of actual countries.[13] Much misery was caused by a single minded set of policy prescriptions that were not well grounded in the larger context for development.

Many development analysts have identified "traps" that have caused Africa's woes. Collier, in *The Bottom Billion* says that conflict, poor governance, either a surplus or deficit of natural resources and being landlocked are the reasons for Africa's poor performance. These are all important variables but it is also important to remember that in Sub-Saharan Africa, economic growth was negative every year during the decade of the 1980s. This was at a time of rapid population growth. During this decade, the rains also failed. Since agriculture in most of Sub-Saharan Africa is still rain fed, not based on irrigation, the combination of negative economic growth and rapid population growth, with the decline of the agricultural sector, explains much of the poverty in this region.

Growth with Strong States: Asia and Pro-Poor Growth Strategies

While the 1980s were called the lost decade for Latin American and Sub-Saharan Africa, it was becoming clear that a different development model was emerging in East Asia as the data for several countries showed remarkable progress in accelerating growth and reducing poverty. For the East Asian countries, the title of a World Bank publication, *The East Asian Miracle: Economic Growth and Public Policy* captured how these societies had succeeded in rebuilding their economies which had been devastated after World War II.

While there are major differences between East and South East Asia on the one hand (China, Indonesia, Thailand and the Philippines) and South Asia (India, Pakistan, Bangladesh and Sri Lanka) and perhaps even more fundamental differences between people living in rural compared to urban areas, the progress during these decades in improving human well-being is unsurpassed by any other regions of the developing world.[14]

In the early 1970s, over half of the people in East, South and Southeast Asia were poor. By 1990 this had fallen to a third and by 2002 to 21.5%. Literacy increased from 47% to over 67% and life expectancy on average improved from 54.3 to 66.6 years. What are the factors that led to these remarkable improvements? Economic growth was a major contributor. However, the initial conditions of most of these countries, especially East and South East were more equitable than Latin America or Sub-Saharan Africa so that when these countries began to grow, growth led to a reduction in poverty.

These countries had invested heavily in improving the basic health and education of their populations, so when economic growth increased, the benefits of that growth were more widely distributed.[15] Fertility levels also dropped substantially during these periods, (in China through draconian population policies.)

The East Asian countries encouraged technology transfer, including foreign direct investment (FDI) that embodied advanced technology, as well as the technology that launched the Green Revolution that increased agricultural yields and reduced hunger and malnutrition. Because poverty is often the highest in rural areas, improving agricultural productivity reduced inequality as well as poverty. Finally, unlike the Latin America and Sub-Saharan Asia, these Asian countries had very high rates of savings. This allowed them to generate their own capital for investment so they did not experience the debt problems of the 1980s. The lessons from these countries development strategies are powerful:

1. Initial infrastructure and human capital conditions matter. The distribution of land, access to basic education and health

care as well as credit shape the equity and inclusiveness of the growth path.

2. Education, health care and gender equity matter. The World Bank's East Asia study concluded "two thirds of growth in the 1965-80 period could be explained by growth in physical and human capital, of which primary education growth was considered the single most important contributor and secondary school enrolment the third important after physical investment." A more recent study concluded that progress in health and nutrition in East and Southeast Asia (less so in South Asia) are also critical factors contributing to the overall success in this region. The results from East Asia and the Pacific on gender equity demonstrate that both improving women's lives contribute to economic growth and also make it more participatory.

3. Investments in infrastructure such as roads and electricity are essential variables contributing to growth as well as poverty reduction. When poor people can access schools and health clinics as well as get their products to markets more easily, their lives are improved and the economy grows.

4. A stable macro economy and access to credit for the poor are key prerequisites for sustainable economic growth as well as reducing poverty.

5. The government bureaucracy needs to be based on merit, not patronage, and

6. The ability to adapt and utilize new technologies is essential for competitiveness in an era of globalization and rapid technological change.

The Asian strategy, while reducing poverty and increasing growth, is not without problems. It has also led to serious environmental degradation, especially in China, as well as increasing income inequality, in particular between urban and rural areas. China's rapid economic growth, fueled by coal, has increased national and global air and water pollution. Moreover, China remains a deeply authoritarian government. The East Asian miracle crashed in the late 1990s as an economic crisis spread throughout Asia. In its wake, scholars began to understand that high levels of corruption and weak institutions were common throughout the region.[16]

1990: Development as Freedom and Protecting the Environment

As the Cold War crumbled along with the Berlin wall in 1989, the motivation for foreign aid based on alignment with the Western bloc also ended. The failure of the policy prescriptions embedded in the Washington consensus led the World Bank, IMF, USAID and other development institutions to conclude that the problems were not necessarily associated with the policies but rather with the institutions in developing countries.

Reforming the institutions of state power and supporting good governance and eventually decentralization, took center stage and remains a key component of most World Bank and bilateral donor programs. How governments can become more effective and accountable became the priority for international donors as well as policy makers in the developing world.

Good governance was the manta that resulted. While there is no commonly accepted definition of good governance,[17] the United Nations defines it as the "exercise of political, economic and administrative authority in the management of a country's affairs." There are several interlinked concepts that define how institutional structures are established that increase the potential for citizens to influence policy effectively and hold governments accountable for their actions. Good governance generally includes four dimensions:

Accountability: Holding governments responsible and protecting against corruption. This can be accomplished through elections when individuals have the freedom and knowledge to evaluate government policies and base their vote on this analysis.

Technical capability: Do government personnel have the skills and knowledge necessary to implement policy? The East Asian societies emphasized the importance of merit-based bureaucracies and left many important decisions to these bureaucrats. In many parts of the world now, especially in the US being a bureaucrat has pejorative connotation. Yet how can good government policies be developed and implemented without people being educated and trained?

Rule of Law: An independent judiciary and predictable rule of law is necessary for sustained growth of the economy and civil society and human rights.

Transparency: Ensuring that the decision processes of government are open to all. In open societies, with freedom of speech and a vibrant free press, government decisions can be debated and evaluated. In the era of the Internet it is harder to hide what governments are doing, although China and other authoritarian governments have succeeded to some extent in preventing citizens from having access to information.

While there is much overlap between notions of democracy and those of governance, good governance is not synonymous with democracy. Political scientists agree that a democratic political system has four defining characteristics:

- A competitive system of elections
- Established and open processes for making policy decisions
- Institutional channels which facilitate participation
- Institutional protections for citizens to ensure safe political participation.

Much has been written about the relationships between democracy and governance and democracy and economic growth.[18] The literature is still inconclusive on the first relationship between democracy and growth but it is clear that it is more likely that a democracy or democratic political system will have at least some of the characteristics of a good governance system such as the rule of law and accountability.

It is possible to have a democratic system, however that has poor governance policies just as it is possible to have some of the characteristics of good governance without having a democratic political system in place. There is also no clear-cut relationship between democracy, governance and growth. The successful Asian societies were not democratic in early growth periods but exhibited many characteristics of good governance.

The ability to hold leaders accountable, which occurs in a democracy has come to be seen a universal human right. A democratic, multi-party political system, with free and fair elections and broad protection of human rights, is the common conceptualization of democracy.

In the late 1980s new actors called by various names—civil society organizations, non-profit and non-governmental actors, began to proliferate. In the last two decades the importance of these intermediate private/public organizations in promoting democracy and economic development has been increasingly recognized. The literature on these organizations suggests that an effective, functioning civil society can increase grassroots participation in the political process, provide voice and empowerment to members, compel governments to be more open, responsive and accountable, and provide important services, especially to the poor. This increased accountability can contribute to the rule of law and better-managed governments, which can support and encourage both democracy and civil society.[19]

Civil society organizations cannot flourish where the right to assemble is not guaranteed. In fact the ability of these organizations to function effectively depends on a human rights environment that supports freedom of speech. Finally improved human rights, which involve the rights of due process and rights to assemble, the ability to speak and petition the government are key components of democratic societies. Human rights are not possible without the rule of law and freedom of speech.

Bringing Government Closer to People

At the end of the twentieth century, as the state led model dissolved under the pressures of globalization and failed economic policies, governments around the world began to decentralize and redistribute power, and in some cases authority and resources to local governments. The motivations for this movement are many and mixed: to bring government "closer to the people" and to make leaders more accountable, to protect individual liberties and check the power of the central government, to build representative government, to identify and satisfy citizen demands for goods and services through improve service delivery and to educate people in weak states about democracy.[20]

The cross-country evidence on the relationship between decentralization, democracy and poverty reduction is mixed. Some research has shown that decentralization can lead to increased corruption as local elites capture power and resources. Moreover, without sufficient financial resources services may not be improved and a broadening of economic and social disparities can result.

While scholars have noted that decentralized governance is not necessarily better than other forms of governance in holding leaders' accountable and improving people's lives,[21] the move to bring government closer to the people, as well as the development of new measures and indices of human development were two of the most important developments in the late 1990s.[22] This is due in great part to the release of a seminal book by Nobel laureate Amartya Sen who said the development is primarily about people having more of a say in their lives.

Development as Freedom

A focus on whether individuals lives were improving, on ensuring the development of human capacities,[23] rather than solely on whether an economy was growing became prominent with the release of the first UNDP Report on Human Development in 1990 and the Human Development Index. The originators of the human development approach and the human development index, Mahbub ul Haq, Paul Streeten, and Amartya Sen said the goal of the human development approach was simply about putting people at the center of the analysis. "After many decades of development, we are rediscovering the obvious—that people are both the means and the end of development. Human development puts people back at the centre stage," said Streeten.[24]

Mahbub ul Haq, both political and policy maker was disillusioned with the single-minded focus on economic growth: "After the Second World War," ul Haq said,

> An obsession grew with economic growth models and national income accounts. People as the agents of change and of development were often forgotten . . . the late 1980s were ripe for a counter-offensive. It was becoming obvious in several countries that human lives were shriveling even as economic production was expanding.[25]

The Human Development paradigm that emerged from the writings of these pioneers is interdisciplinary and normative.[26] Drawing on the long history of political thought that includes Kant, Rousseau and Rawls this approach focuses on issues of justice and social equity. The end of development, according to this framework is to expand people's freedom and capabilities in all areas: economic, political, social and cultural. The Human Development Index (HDI) that resulted from these original efforts, a composite index that measures life expectancy, education and gross domestic product, has become an important counter-weight to measuring development simply using GDP or GNI.[27]

An essential component of the human development framework is empowerment. Empowerment, according to Haq, includes, "a political democracy in which people can influence decisions about their lives . . . so that real governance is brought to the doorstep of every person. It means that all members of civil society, particularly non-governmental organizations, are participating fully in making and implementing decisions."[28]

Sen's capability approach is a normative framework that defines development as freedom.[29] The goal of development should be to expand the freedom that poor people have to enjoy "valuable beings and doings." Development, says Sen, should be evaluated in terms of the expansion of people's capabilities to lead the kind of life they value. The expansion of these capabilities depends both on the ability to participate freely in decision-making and on the provision of basic goods. People need both—the resources for improving their lives but also the ability to make the choices that matter to them. Expanding choices and resources for individuals should be the goal of development, according to Sen's approach.[30]

The approach forces an important question when evaluating development performance: do people have the freedom to lead the kind of life they determine as important, and the resources necessary to meet these self determined values. People are the ends, not the means of development and through political participation should be able to express what they value, make their own choices, and have access to the resources to meet these goals.

Much of the debate about whether countries are democratic or not has focused on the institutions and mechanisms of government, especially whether elections are free and fair and whether civil liberties are present. These formal institutions of a democratic society are essential if governance is to be democratic but miss how democracies function, and the extent to which individuals are able to participate and influence decision-making at all levels. The key question to ask is whether the institutions empower citizens to participate in decision-making and whether the decisions matter in improving their lives. Democracy is stronger some argue when it leads to improvements in basic needs, reduces poverty and increases access to higher education and culture.

Democracy's accomplishments—or not—should be part of the analysis. However, few of our definitions and measurements of democracy are this broad. Instead, they have been simplistic and at a low level of analysis. Some are even binary: democratic, not democratic. We have failed to look deeply in societies to answer this simple but essential question: do individuals have the ability to influence decisions about issues important to improving their lives and have these decisions led to improvements?[31]

At the dawn of the 21st century local governments in Latin America, Asia and parts of Sub-Saharan Africa, including Rwanda began a process of shifted resources and authority from the central to local governments. Have these experiments led to increased democratic governance, to expanded capabilities and improvements in the lives of the poor?

Sustaining the Environment

As the twentieth century ended, an influential commission released a report that added a significant dimension to the definition of development. The Brundtland Commission Report (World Commission on Environment and Development, 1987) began to document the impact of industrialization on the global environment, and that sustainable development, "meets the needs of the present without compromising the ability of future generations to meet their own needs."

We have come to recognize that the classical economic assumption that economic growth can continue unconstrained by the carrying capacity of the ecosphere, once tenable when only a small proportion of human societies experienced rapid and sustained growth, is no longer sustainable when all the human societies on earth are striving for rapid growth to develop.

Economic production depends upon the ecosystem as a source for new raw material inputs and as a sink to absorb the waste, byproducts, and recycled outputs of the production. For development to be sustainable, in the definition of the Brundtland commission,[32] it must not interfere with the ecosystem's capacity to sustain the productive activity of future generations. Sustainable development minimizes the use of nonrenewable natural resources, the emission of wastes and pollutants, and the impact in general on the existing biodiversity and ecological processes of the ecosystem.

It is possible, in theory and increasingly in practice, for economic development to enable a human being to achieve at the same time both a higher material standard of living and a lessened environmental impact. This requires policies that: 1) regulate and raise the costs of resource use and pollution, favoring labor intensity over resource or capital intensity; 2) encourage environmentally friendly technological change and openness to the best environmental technology globally available; 3) provide a better public infrastructure (water, sewerage, and power systems); and 4) speed the transition from the high-impact primary sector of the economy (farming, forestry, fishing, and mining) through the higher value-added secondary sector (processing and manufacturing) to the lowest-impact, highest productivity service sectors (the production of new information, knowledge, communications, and entertainment).

Role of Information Technology

Students of modernization and development have long examined the impact of science and technology on development. The information technology revolution has caused such worldwide change that it is challenging to study its impact. As a result, few development studies have yet to understand or analyze how new information and communication technologies allow poor countries to leapfrog past stages of development.[33] In education, health care, economic growth, and political participation, Internet-based technologies as well as cell phones, are playing key positive roles. They broaden the depth and scope of information in a society, and when this information is transformed into knowledge through education and learning, becomes useful knowledge that can improve lives and societies. Most importantly, as we have seen throughout history, technological advances are one of the primary drivers of economic growth.

The Dawn of the 21st Century

In 2000, the development community came together to codify a set of standards for evaluating whether countries are "on track." The Millennium Development goals were the results. Widely hailed as the appropriate and essential economic and social goals that developing countries should strive to reach by 2015, they are poorly designed, incomplete, have serious methodical and conceptual problems, and are negatively biased against Africa. Yet almost every country, including Rwanda, has developed statistical capacity to measure progress against these eight goals, and global assistance is dependent upon countries efforts to reach them.[34] Our analysis of Rwanda's progress and development includes a review a progress towards meeting these goals.

Table 2.1
The Eight Millennium Development Goals

1. Eradicate extreme poverty and hunger
2. Achieve universal primary education
3. Promote gender equality and empower women
4. Reduce child mortality
5. Improve maternal health
6. Combat HIV/AIDS malaria and other disease
7. Ensure environmental sustainability
8. Develop a global partnership for development

Lessons Learned: An Evidence-Based Framework

After six decades of development study, programs and projects, how can we best define development and what is the best evidence about how best to improve the quality of peoples lives? While there is no agreed upon definition of development, we propose that a sustainable society is one that is economically inclusive, environmentally sustainable, socially just, and participatory.

We will judge Rwanda's progress by asking the following five questions, for all of which there is real evidence to evaluate.

1. Are citizens participating freely in decisions that shape their lives and has the country made progress in establishing democracy?

Specifically, has Rwanda made progress in developing decision-making institutions and structures that are inclusive and that allow all citizens to participate regardless of ethnic background, and make choices about what they value?

2. Is access to primary, secondary and tertiary education widespread?

Education improves individual lives, opens up economic and social opportunities, and is the basis for becoming a modern society. Rwanda's leaders think that the best way to move from an agriculturally based economy to an information and knowledge-based society is though widespread access and use of ICT. In Rwanda, is education available, and improving? How far along is Rwanda in using information and communications technologies?

3. Are women able to participate in all levels of society?

Gender equity is a basic right and instrumental in improving a society. Scholars have been able to demonstrate for many decades that economic investments in girls and women have a far greater impact, especially on children and families, than similar investments in men. When women are educated, infant and child mortality is reduced, female fertility declines, and over time family and national income improves. When women participate in government, corruption may be reduced. How involved are women in Rwanda's government, decision-making structures, and educational system?

4. Is access to health care, including reproductive health care, widespread, in both urban and rural areas?

Social or human development includes improved health care for a population, increased literacy, improved nutrition, adequate shelter, poverty reduction, and improved gender equity and population stability. In many ways these objectives, improving the physical quality of life of all citizens, along with a sustainable environment can be seen as the primary goals of development. Improvements in these indicators also affect other aspects of development. For example, improved literacy and health care lead to productivity improvements, thus to economic growth, and to increased participation in society and the labor force. How much has health care improved in Rwanda during the past fifteen years?

5. Is economic growth pro-poor?

The lessons of the Asian tigers are important models for economic growth. The goal of economic development is to increase growth but in such a way that the benefits of growth are equitably distributed.[34] A healthy growing economy also requires strong macro-economic management, which includes a sustainable balance of payments and sound monetary and fiscal policies. None of these economic policies can be effectively implemented unless the government has the capability (and willingness) to manage them. Has economic growth in Rwanda helped the poor? Has growth succeeded in reducing food insecurity? What is the impact of economic growth on the environment in Rwanda?

It seems to us that these five questions are ones that we could ask of all countries, questions that are susceptible to investigation and the gathering of hard evidence. This is what we propose to do now for the case of Rwanda, in hopes that we can learn something valuable from its experience and singular accomplishments. Each chapter that follows summarizes the progress and assesses the challenges remaining.

Notes

1. An excellent review of the major development ideas of the past six decades can be found in Richard Jolly. L. Emmerij and Thomas Weiss, "The Power of UN Ideas: Lessons from the first 60 Years." *The United Nations Intellectual History Project*. London: Grundy and Northedge, 2005.

2. World Bank. *World Development Report 2008: Agriculture for Development*. Washington, D.C.: The World Bank, 2008.

3. See Rodrick, Dani, ed. *In Search of Prosperity: Analytic Narratives on Economic Growth*. Princeton: Princeton University Press, 2003, and Rodrick, Dani. "Rethinking Growth Policies in the Developing World." The Luca d'Agliano Lecture in Development Economics Delivered October 8, 2004.

4. See ILO, 1976.

5. Paul Streeten, *First Things First: Meeting Basic Human Needs in the Developing Countries*. New York: Oxford University Press.

6. Nancy Birdsall, Nancy "Population Growth: Its Magnitude and Implications for Development." *Finance and Development* (1984): 10-15.

7. See R. Bulatao, *Reducing Fertility in Developing Countries: A Review of Determinants and Policy Levers*. Washington, D.C. The World Bank, 1984. Also see the journal, *Population and Development Review*.

8. See World Bank. *Engendering Development Through Gender Equality in Rights, Resources and Voice*. Washington, D.C. The World Bank, 2001.

9. Amar Hamoudi and Jeffrey D. Sachs. "Economic Consequences of Health Status: A Review of the Evidence." Harvard University Center for International Development Working Paper No. 30 (December 1999) 1-25. and World Bank, 1993 and 2001.

10. For information on the "Global Burden of Disease" and the DALY measurement see the World Health Organization website at www.who.int/healthinfo/global_burdendisease/en/index.html.

11. Haddad, Wadi. *Education and Development: Evidence for New Priorities*. Washington, D.C.: The World Bank, 1990.

12. For one summary see, Jeffrey Sachs, ed. *Developing Country Debt and Economic Performance*. Chicago: University of Chicago Press, 1989.

13. See Rodrick, 2004.

14. See Kaplinsky, Raphel and Dirk Messner. "Introduction: The Impact of Asian Drivers on the Developing World." *World Development* Vol. 36, No. 2 (2007): 197-209, and Lin, Justin Yifu. "Development Strategies for Inclusive Growth in Developing Asia." *Asian Development Review* Vol. 21, No. 2 (2004): 1-27.

15. Chatterjee, Shiladitya. "Poverty Reduction Strategies—Lessons from the Asian and Pacific Region on Inclusive Development." *Asian Development Review* Vol. 22 No. 1 (2005): 12-44.

16. Joseph Stiglitz, ed. *Rethinking the East Asian Miracle*. New York: Oxford University Press, 2001.

17. Marilee Grindle, "Good Enough Governance Revisited." *Development Policy Review* Vol. 25 No. 5 (2007): 553-574 and Alpha Diedhiou, "Governance for Development: Understanding the Concept/Reality Linkages." *Journal of Human Development* Vol. 8 No. 1 (March, 2007): 23-38, and Martin Doorknobs, "'Good Governance: The Metamorphosis of a Policy Metaphor." *Journal of International Affairs* Vol. 57, No. 1 (2003): 3-17.

18. See Barro, Robert J. "Democracy and Growth." *Journal of Economic Growth* (March 1996): 1-27.

19. Indrajit Roy, "Civil Society and Good Governance: Re-Conceptualizing the Interface. *World Development* Vol. 36, No. 4 (2008): 677-705.

20. Philip Oxhorn, Joseph S. Tulchin and Andrew D. Selee. *Decentralization, Democratic Governance and Civil Society in Comparative Perspective: Africa, Asia and Latin America*. Baltimore: Johns Hopkins University Press, 2004, Merilee Grindle, Grindle, *Going Local: Decentralization, Democratization and the Promise of Good Governance*. Princeton: Princeton University Press, 2007. G. Cheema, G. Shabbir and Dennis Rondinelli, eds. *Decentralizing Governance: Emerging Concepts and Practices*. Washington, D.C.: Brookings Institution Press, 2007, Olowu, Dele and James Wunsch. *Local Governance in Africa: The Challenges of Democratic Decentralization*. Boulder: Lynne Reinner Publishers, 2004.

21. Treisman, Daniel. *The Architecture of Government: Rethinking Political Decentralization*. Cambridge: Cambridge University Press, 2007.

22. See Philip Oxhorn, Joseph S. Tulchin and Andrew D. Selee. *Decentralization, Democratic Governance and Civil Society in Comparative Perspective: Africa, Asia and Latin America*. Baltimore: Johns Hopkins University Press, 2004; Cheema, G. Shabbir and Dennis Rondinelli, eds. *Decentralizing Governance: Emerging Concepts and Practices*. Washington, D.C.: Brookings Institution Press, 2007 and Merilee Grindle, *Going Local: Decentralization, Democratization and the Promise of Good Governance*. Princeton: Princeton University Press, 2007.

23. Evans, Peter "Collective Capabilities, Culture and Amartya Sen's Development as Freedom." *Studies in Comparative International Development* Vol. 37, No. 2 (Summer 2002): 54-60 for a good summary of this approach.

24. See Streeten, 1981.

25. Mahbub ul Haq, *Reflections on Human Development*. New York: Oxford University Press, 1995 P. 25.

26. Gustav Ranis, Francis Stewart and Emma Samman. "Human Development: Beyond the Human Development Index." *Journal of Human Development* Vol. 7. No. 3 (November 2006): 323-357. Amaryta Sen, "Development Thinking at the Beginning of the 21st Century." Paper Presented at the Conference on Development Thinking and Practice, Inter-American Development Bank, Washington D.C. 3-5 September, 1996 and Amartya Sen, *Development as Freedom*. New York: Anchor Books, 2000.

27. Ranis, Gustav, Francis Stewart and Emma Samman. "Human Development: Beyond the Human Development Index." *Journal of Human Development* Vol. 7. No. 3 (November 2006): 323-357.

28. Mahbub ul Haq, *Reflections on Human Development*. New York: Oxford University Press, 1995 P. 22.

29. Sabina Alkire, "Why the Capability Approach?" *Journal of Human Development* Vol. 6. No 1. (2005): 115-133.

30. Srinivasan, Sharath. "No Democracy without Justice: Amaryta Sen's unfinished business with the capability approach." Doctoral research, University of Oxford.

31. Crocker, David A. "Deliberative Participation in Local Development." *Journal of Human Development* Vol. 8 No. 3 (November, 2007): 431-55.

32. See United Nations *Report of the World Commission on Environment and Development: Our Common Future. Document A/42/427.* New York: The United Nations, 1987, commonly refereed to as the Brundtland Report because the Commission was chaired by the former Prime Minister of Norway, Dr. Brundtland.

33. Vitro, Robert ed. *The Knowledge Economy in Development: Perspectives for Effective Partnerships*. Washington, D.C.: Inter-American Development Bank, 2005, and Misuraca, Gianluca. *E-Governance in Africa: From Theory to Action*. Trenton, N.J.: Africa World Press, 2007.

34. Republic of Rwanda, National Institute of Statistics: *Rwanda Development Indicators 2006*, Kigali, 2008.

35. See Nanak Kakwani and Ernesto Pernia. "What is Pro-Poor Growth?" *Asian Development Review* Vol. 18, No. 1 (2000): 1-16.

Chapter Three

Are Citizens Participating Freely in Decision-Making?

On July 4, 1994, the forces of the Rwandan Patriotic Front (RPF) defeated the genocidal Habyarimana government. Close to a million people were dead. The country was in ruins. The killers were fleeing toward Zaire, where they would re-arm and continue the fighting for over a decade. After ignoring the genocide, the international community rushed resources to the NGOs supporting these so-called refugees. The already fragile infrastructure was destroyed. Schools, hospitals and homes were in ruins. Agriculture was destroyed. Neighbors hated neighbors, families were torn apart. Priests had killed members of their congregations. The social, economic, physical and emotional fabric was destroyed.

How did Rwanda begin to rebuild? It began with a question.

We only asked one question: "What caused the disunity among us?" Each community was broken up into five groups. The survivors of the genocide were in one group; the returnees from Tanzania, Zaire, Uganda and other countries were in another. The 1959 returnees constituted another group, those who had stayed in their location another, and finally the elite and highly educated were in another group. We told people three things:

1. There is to be no revenge.
2. Share what you have with the rest.
3. We are going to discuss and dialogue.

We knew that everyone was afraid. In fact, fear and insecurity are what everyone shared. The results were surprising. After a long process of discussions and meetings four reasons emerged:

- *Inda Nini, which literally means big stomach—that people had been selfish and the nation had been misgoverned.*
- *Poverty, ignorance and colonialism were the other top answers.*

There was no civil society; so two people were elected from each of the five groups to discuss the problem more and to come up with solutions. We were trying to create a process that people could trust. Everything was written down and tabulated. At the end of this long process one old man asked me: "Why didn't you ask this question before we killed each other?" The process was as important as the answers. People began talking to each other again. It was not easy but it was the beginning of the dialogue.[1]

From that first question, and those long dialogues that began as the country was in ruins, a model of governance and democracy is emerging that is based on the rule of law, separation of powers, democratic decentralization, unity and reconciliation, and accountability. From a failed state, a capable state has emerged that has developed a participatory, democratic process for all citizens, including and especially the poor, youth, women, the disabled, and even those who participated in the genocide.

After over a decade of work and research in the country, attending Parliamentary committee meetings, sitting in on judicial hearings, observing needs assessments at the local level (Ubudehe) and trials, watching and participating in national dialogue discussions, interviewing over 100 legislators, judges, educators, health professionals, mayors, Ministers, Senators and the President, as well as interviewing Rwandan professionals living outside the country, it is clear to us that Rwanda is making dramatic progress toward a building a society based on inclusiveness, accountability, the rule of law and is giving voice to the poor.[2]

Rwanda's evolution in building political institutions must be examined and evaluated in a broad perspective: The world ignored the genocide, then once it had been stopped by the Rwanda Patriotic Army (RPA) the major powers and donor community turned their attention to supporting the organizers and perpetrators as they fled to Eastern Congo.[3]

The French, threatened by the possibility of an English-speaking regime taking power, and closely aligned with the Habyarimana regime, intervened during the genocide. In June 1994 they established what was called Zone Turquoise in southwestern Rwanda with the pretext of protecting Tutsi (few were alive by then) but which allowed the genocidiares to escape to Zaire. The French denied their involvement in supporting the Habyarimana regime and from the beginning criticized the new Rwandan rulers as a way to distance themselves from their own history and actions.[4]

The Catholic Church in Rwanda was deeply involved in building the Hutu Power ideology that allowed the genocide to occur.[5] Catholic leaders strongly voiced their own innocence and proclaimed their concern about the RPA. The new leaders were on their own.

Within the country this was the legacy: for three decades an elected government of the majority had tried to first exclude then exterminate the minority. In Rwanda democracy had come to mean annihilation of the Tutsis by the ethnic majority, the Hutus. From the 1960 elections at independence to the Habyarimana election in 1988, elections had reinforced this notion.

President Habyarimana, elected in 1973 had modeled his party, the National Revolutionary Movement for Development (MRND) after the North Korean Communist Party. Every Rwandan became a member at birth and the country was ruled until the genocide began in 1994 with political intimidation and terror. The Tutsis were excluded entirely from the political process. Massacres of Tutsis, which had started after the Belgians turned power over to the Hutus in 1962, accelerated in 1990. The political party at independence, the Democratic Republican Movement-Parmehutu (MDR-Parmehutu) began the repression of Tutsi's and suppression of opposition. By 1990 the media controlled the political space and broadcast the hate message of Hutu Power. Hutu Power claimed that the RPF would kill all Hutus if their "invasion" was successful.

All political structures: the electoral system, the legislature, the judiciary, the executive branch and the media were completely compromised and without legitimacy. It would take the new leadership over a decade to build legitimacy and trust in these essential institutions.

There is no single agreed upon blueprint for building a society based on democratic governance, especially one that had thirty years of a history based on an ideology of hate and ethnic division, that resulted in genocide. Moreover, few countries in modern times have been confronted

with the carnage facing Rwanda's leaders in July of 1994, as well as the
continuing threats to human security. "I returned to Kigali in July, 1994.
There was nothing left standing and only bodies on the street," said
Professor Kimenyi from California State University in Sacramento. From
that daunting period, new institutions and democratic principles have
been established and are evolving that offer progress and hope not only
for the citizens of Rwanda but for other post-conflict societies as well.

In Rwanda today, a constitution is in place that guarantees separation
of powers for the first time in the country's history. An independent
judiciary is in place and Gacaca trials, representing one of the greatest
legal challenges in history, are underway. National and local elections
have been held. An Ombudsman and auditor general's office have been
established to ensure accountability and reduce corruption. As a result,
numerous senior political figures have been jailed. Recently, in several
international rankings, including a World Bank governance index, Rwanda
has ranked as one of the least corrupt countries in the region, and most
improved in the rule of law.[6]

Through processes called Ubudehe and Imihigo, poor people are
deeply involved in solving their own problems through representative
democratic processes that hold leaders accountable through performance
contracts. Ubudehe, an inclusive and participatory process and system is
unlike anything else in the world. It is a way for all, including and especially the poor, to have input into a decision making process that ulti-
mately can improve their lives. Imihigos holds leaders accountable. These
old customs—adapted for the 21st century—empower people and give
them hope that their lives can be improved.

In the midst of physical and emotional ruin, people began talking to
each other again and it has not stopped in fifteen years. A great deal of
the success of present day Rwanda is because of decisions made at the
conclusion of the genocide in July, 1994 toward reconciliation, policies
enacted by the legislature, the development of an independent judiciary
and a strong and clear vision that emerged from the President. It is a
powerful reminder of the importance of accountable, visionary, and knowledgeable leaders and structures. Rwanda reminds us that leadership and
policy at the local, regional and national level matter. They matter a
great deal.

How did this structure and process originate and evolve? In part it is
a story that highlights the importance of dialogue and participation in
rebuilding a country that had lost its way. "When people are oppressed

or reduced to the culture of silence, they do not participate in their own humanization. Conversely when they participate, thereby becoming active subjects of knowledge and action, they begin to construct their properly human history and engage in processes of authentic development."[7] Rwanda is an example of how oppressed people not only were silent, but also became killers, and how through meaningful participation in constructing their own lives, are being reborn.

This positive story of progress in political development is a story that few outside Rwanda are aware of and some, especially genocide deniers, are resisting. Genocide deniers continue to expose a hate ideology both within the country and around the world, including in the US, Europe and Canada. Major human rights organizations reject acknowledging Rwanda's progress in providing security for all Rwandans, developing democratic structures and encouraging political participation.

In a recent volume on justice and reconstruction in Rwanda, the editors discuss the rise of revisionism and its impact on our understanding of the genocide and post genocide situation in Rwanda:

> Equally troubling is the growing revisionism regarding the genocide. A range of voices from Hutu ideologies to Western academics has grown louder in recent years, claiming either there was no genocide of Tutsi in 1994 or that there is little substantive difference between crimes against Tutsi and those perpetrated against Hutu by the RPF and Tutsi civilians. Genocide revisionism is not new; as displayed by the host of deniers of the holocaust, which has prompted the passing of anti-denial legislation in many countries. In the Rwandan case, genocide deniers have a variety of motivations: scholars pursuing the latest academic fads that revel in "alternative narratives," no matter how spurious or morally questionable; genocidiares seeking to deflect attention from their crimes' and critics of the current RPF government who try to connect alleged RPF atrocities in 1994 to unrelated concerns with its current policies.[8]

This chapter describes the history and development of political processes from 1994 to 2009, with an emphasis on the period from 2003-08. It evaluates progress and discusses challenges in establishing democratic institutions and processes, justice and reconciliation, and human rights. While a literature is emerging about what happened before and during the genocide,[9] little has been written so far about this early period[10] so the majority of this section depends on extensive interviews, primary documents, and donor documents, including those from the IMF, UNDP, World Bank and USAID.

The Transition Period 1994-2003: Security Challenges

In the months following the liberation of the county by the RPA establishing security and dealing with the economic and social consequences of the genocide dominated the new leadership.

"I spent the first six months burying people," said Rose Kabuye, the first Mayor of the city of Kigali. From 1994-96 the country's leaders focused on stabilizing the country, repatriating refugees, and trying to provide for basic necessities such as shelter, food and water. "There was nothing to eat," said Bonaventure. "We all started growing what food we could." "There was no electricity or running water in Kigali until late 1994," said Tom Ndahiro, a journalist and editor of a Rwandan newspaper from 1994-99 who went on to be elected by Parliament to become one of the country's first human rights commissioners, in charge of Civil and Political Rights. He gathered primary documents while the genocide was occurring, pertaining to the involvement of the French, the Catholic Church as well as the Habyarimana government. "Most of the infrastructure was destroyed," said Ndahiro. "The little remaining, especially the houses, was soon taken over by international NGOs who caused a great deal of inflation. By 1995 most of Kigali had power again. Members of the new government did it mainly by themselves."

Security and stability were the priorities during these early years. The majority of the genocide organizers had fled to the Congo and were reorganizing and re-arming in the refugee camps, to continue the genocide. The international community, at first not understanding what was occurring in the camps, responded generously with close to $1 million a day in assistance for the refugees.[11] The new government, facing unimaginable challenges, had to rely on its own meager resources.

Military and political control was highly centralized in the first few years. The security situation was extremely volatile. While the RPF captured Kigali city in July 1994, the war continued in the northwest. Cross border raids from what was then Zaire (now the Democratic Republic of the Congo) into eastern Rwanda began in late 1994 and continued through 1996 when Rwanda invaded Zaire in order to stop the incursions. During this entire period the cross border raids from Zaire targeted genocide survivors and Hutus who cooperated with the government in rebuilding the country.[12]

The Rwandan army aligned and supported Yoweri Museveni's in Uganda. Many Rwandan leaders had been senior leaders in the Ugandan army. Eventually with the support of Angolan and Zimbabwean troops, they succeeded in ousting Zaire's dictator Mobutu Sese Seko, in 1997, and putting in power Laurent Kabila. Mobuto had long been aligned and supported by the United States government during the Cold War. The new President initially supported his regional backers, but the alignment was short-lived. Soon after the Kabila government was installed in Kinshasa, in May 1997, Kabila began arming the Interhamwe and former Rwandan Armed Forces (ex-FAR). A new war began in Eastern Congo that raged until 2002, leaving close to a million dead in Eastern Congo. This second mass killing was a result of the conflict but also because of starvation and disease. Why the international community neglected this desperate situation and why the intervention, when it came was so minimal, is worthy of closer investigation.

While the security within the country remained very precarious, on July 17, less than two weeks after the liberation of the country, RPA leaders published a document outlining the basic principles for the transition government. The new state institutions and governing principles would be based on the previously negotiated Arusha Accords, the Habyarimana government has agreed to a set of principles for power sharing that. The RPF, "pledged commitment to the rule of law, the construction of a national army open to all Rwandans, the sitting of a government of national unity based on an inclusive coalition of political forces. They also affirmed the legitimacy of the Constitution of 1991 as well as the Arusha Accords as the fundamental rules for governing the nation."[13] With the daunting security situation, political control was tight. A Government of National Unity was formed under the Rwandan Patriotic Front (RPF) with membership from other parties not directly implicated in the genocide.

One of the most immediate problems facing the new government was how to deal with those who had participated in the genocide. Soon after the genocide ended, the United Nations Security Council adopted Resolution 955 that established the International Criminal Tribunal for Rwanda. Its charge was to "prosecute persons responsible for genocide and other serious violations of international humanitarian law committed in the territory of Rwanda and Rwandan citizens responsible for genocide and other such violations committed in the territory of neighboring States, between 1 January 1994 and 31 December 1994. . . ."[14]

Most of the organizers had fled the country but many of the killers were either in refugee camps in Zaire, or had fled to neighboring countries. The prisons were overflowing with the killers. The UN, initially with support from the new Rwandan government, chose to set up a tribunal to try the organizers of the genocide outside the country, in Arusha, Tanzania. Quickly, a contentious relationship developed with the International Criminal Tribunal for Rwanda or ICTR that contended justice could not be served within the country, and the Rwandan leaders who felt strongly that justice required that the killers be tried where the survivors could witness the hearings.

The Beginnings

Four government institutions were created in the summer of 1994: The Transitional Government, the Transitional National Assembly, the judiciary and the Presidency of the Republic. This first government included all parties who had not participated in the genocide. Initially designed to end in 1999; the transition period was extended until July 19, 2003 when the new constitution was adopted.

The Transitional National Assembly, or legislature, followed the design of the 1993 Arusha Peace Accords that had been agreed to by the RFF as well as the Habyarimana government. The 74 Members of Parliament were appointed, not elected, based on eight political parties that predated the RPF takeover in 1994. The parties that had been instrumental in designing the genocide, the MDR and MRND were banned.

It is remarkable, that nascent democratic institutions were established at all during this early period of reconstruction. Yet interviews with Members of Parliament who participated in this first Transitional Assembly were consistent in their philosophy: "We had the opportunity to build a country based on tolerance, reconciliation and unity," said Senator Aloysie Inyumba, a member of the Transitional Assembly.

These new legislators worked in a Parliament building that had holes in the walls from the recent fighting, and few of the basic necessities like pencils and paper. Their power came from several laws: the Fundamental Law that included the 1991 constitution, the 1993 Arusha Peace Accords, the 1994 Declaration of the Rwandan Patriotic Front and the 1994 protocol agreement of the Forum of Political Parties.) Additional powers were defines in the "Organic Laws" which were only superseded by the Constitution in importance.[15]

The Arusha Peace Agreements had also stipulated that the five top positions in the country be divided among the different political parties. The Transition Government followed this stipulation: the President of the Republic (RPF), the Prime-Minister (MDR) the National Assembly President (PSD) the Assembly Vice-President (PL) and Assembly Secretary Deputy (PDC) were to be divided different parties. Pasteur Bizimungu became President and General Paul Kagame took the newly created post of Vice-Presidency as well as Minister of Finance. Both represented the RFP. Faustin Twagiramungu, representing the MDR party became first Prime Minister. Political parties were restricted during this transitional period. They could not recruit new members or publicize their activities. No new parties could organize unless approved by the legislature.

From the first days of the Assembly, the Parliamentarians had extensive legal powers to develop laws including the budget of the government. Voting was done by a show of hands, orally or electronically or by secret ballot at the request of a fifth of the Deputies."[16] Significantly, and an early sign of women's commitment to rebuilding Rwandan, a quarter of the new MPs were women. The Assembly powers were expanded considerably in 1997 when they gained the right to adopt the budget as well as the right to question Ministers of the Executive branch.

The legislature began asserting its authority to question the executive branch in 2000. By 2001, the Assembly had held 11 sessions devoted to questioning Ministers and with a vote of two-thirds could censure a Minister forcing a resignation. However the majority of legislation during the transitional period was initiated by the Executive branch. From 1994 until the enactment of the Constitution in 2003, 240 bills were passed with 20 initiated by the MPs.

The early years were extremely challenging for the new legislators. They had few resources. None of the MPs had been members of a government. But they had hope and vision.

The Judiciary

As the country and leaders faced the daunting task of rebuilding and taking the first steps toward reconciliation, the primary question was who would judge those who committed the atrocities. There were few judges left alive. The justice system was destroyed. The army was establishing security and reducing violence but the country could not rebuild without a process and structure for reconciliation and justice. "We were in total shambles in 1994," said Judge Busingye who participated in writing the new laws. "There was nothing. Most of the judges had been killed." Statistics gathered by the Office of the Gacaca Courts show how dire the situation was in 1994, with only 12 prosecutors and 244 judges left in the country.

Table 3.1
Impact of Genocide on the Judiciary

Reference Period	Judges	Prosecutors	Support Staff
Before 1994	758	70	631
November 1994	244	12	137

Source: Republic of Rwanda, *National Service of Gacaca Courts*, February, 2008.

Johnston Busingye, a survivor, lawyer, someone who was deeply involved in rebuilding the justice sector, and who is now President of the High Court in Rwanda, was interviewed extensively for this book. One of us also visited his courtroom on numerous occasions, once when he overturned a government case. He describes what it was like in 1994:

There were no standards, no minimum standards for the judiciary, and no academic standards. There was only incompetence and corruption. One of the main things we had to achieve was independence of (the) judiciary from (the) political structure. The President called a large meeting with teachers, doctors, and professionals. He asked us: "What is the big problem?" Corruption, we said is the issue. "Then how do we solve it?" We had to be open and honest. The Law Commission started after these discussions (in 1999) and did not end until 2001. The commission was given full powers. There were judges, prosecutors and two lawyers. There were no politicians, no army. We were given independence from the Minister of Justice. We were answerable only to Parliament. The Government did not change anything we recommended; it then went to Parliament and we got the finances to pay for it. No one was controlling us—politically or economically. In the first six to seven months the commissions reviewed what we could find on the workings of a good and modern judiciary. We did a study tour of the US, the Netherlands, Norway, South Africa, and Madagascar to look at countries which have had mixed system. We also visited countries that were French colonies based on civil law, and the Netherlands, Denmark and Sweden known for mix of civil and common law. We asked what is best from all these systems that Rwanda can use to make law.[17]

In 1995 then President Pasteur Bizimungu organized an international conference to discuss methods for dealing with the genocidiares. One of the ideas that emerged was the notion of using a traditional process called Gacaca. Gacaca, which in Kinyarwanda means, "grass" is a conflict resolution method that had been used in pre-colonial times to deal with far less serious crimes than murder.

While other ideas were debated at the conference, including using the South African Truth and Reconciliation approach, it was decided to proceed with developing the legislation needed to establish Gacaca in a formal way. The legislation that was passed by the National Assembly, called Organic Law 08/96 established four categories of offenders:

1. The organizers and planners of the genocide
2. Those who had committed murder but were not organizers
3. Those who had committed serious crimes against other persons and
4. Crimes against property.

Part of the legislation included a reduction in penalties for those who confessed. At the outset there was significant international criticism of the Gacaca process, specifically that it failed international standards for a fair trail. William Schabas in "Post Genocide Justice in Rwanda," states that some of the criticisms "were made by lawyers trained in common law jurisdiction, who misunderstood certain aspects of the 'civil law' approach that Rwanda had inherited from Belgium and France. . . . Lawyers trained in common law jurisdiction . . . were shocked at the relative brevity of the trials, the reliance on written evidence and the lack of cross-examination. By contrast, trial lawyers who came from 'civil law' traditions were relatively sanguine and even rather impressed with the proceedings."[18]

There were few alternatives for dealing with this many cases of murder. The justice system was destroyed. Initially the idea of using Gacaca for trying the perpetrators of genocide was rejected. Tharcisse Karugarama, now the Minister of Justice, was one of the people who raised the idea soon after the end of the genocide. "It was totally rejected,"[19] he said. Eventually, Gacaca would become an important tool for reconciliation. A pilot phase began in 2002 but it was not until 2006 that the process was formalized on a nationwide basis.

Even at this early stage of rebuilding, Rwandans turned back to traditional processes that had been used in pre-colonial times. Many of these traditional structures are now embedded in the justice and governance systems. Five indigenous programs and processes have become important in rebuilding and reconciliation.

- Gacaca is the name of the community based trials, (in Kinyarwanda Gacaca means grass) which are now underway for the second-level genocidiares.
- Umuganda: originally a community coming together on a voluntary basis to work on community projects, this has been adapted as the basis for labor-intensive public works projects to create jobs and build incomes.
- Ubudehe is a participatory process developed from a traditional concept of working collectively in agriculture. Ubudehe took place when all social and ethnic groups prepared the fields together before the rains came and the planting season arrived. It now refers to a participatory process of needs assessment, budgeting and planning at the village level, whereby citizens themselves allocate decentralized funds according to village priorities.
- Umusanzu: A tradition for supporting the needy is now used to support educational funds for the poor and is the basis for the "Mutuelle de Santé,' heath initiative.
- Imihigo: Traditional a competitive contest to determine who is best in a community now used to describe the performance-management system of governance that began at the local level.

While many of these practices were present throughout Sub-Saharan Africa in pre-colonial times, the programs in Rwanda are unique in that they draw on the nation's cultural past, and combined with modern legal concepts to build trust, to reconcile, and especially for the poor and illiterate, to build the knowledge and skills necessary in a democratic society.

Human Rights

International human rights organizations began their criticism of the new leaders soon after those same leaders stopped the genocide.[20] Rwanda's response was to develop its own Human Rights Council, which was established in May 1995. Their charge was to investigate human rights abuses as well as implement the international human rights covenants that Rwanda had agreed to including covenants on civil and political rights. "Many people did not know their rights," said Tom Ndahiro one of the first Human Rights Commissioners. "We had to do a lot of monitoring and education."

> In the first 2-3 years after the commission started we found, for example, that people were being detained and held illegally without proper documents. We investigated these cases and started teaching about human rights in the schools. We also worked with the UN High Commissioner for Human Rights who sent a special representative to work with us. There were many issues in the beginning—freedom of expression, detention, and some instances of torture. We had to educate people about human rights and about the covenants Rwanda had signed and ratified. We worked hard until 1999 when there were very few serious cases left. By then mechanisms had been put in place and the plans for the constitution included the human rights principles from these international human rights instruments."[21]

National Unity and Reconciliation Committee (NURC)

The National Unity and Reconciliation Committee (NURC) was also established soon after the government was established in 1994. Its charge was to begin a process of civic education and training sessions (Ingando) that educated and prepared the population for the beginning of the gacaca trials, as well as re-integrated ex-rebels from the Democratic Republic of the Congo.

Conflict Resolution and Building Unity:
Ubudehe to Village Urugwiro

By early 1997, the immediate security threats had been reduced and grass roots discussions and consultations continued.

> After a while, people really wanted to participate. So they were included when we began asking the next question: What are the major problems facing the country. We discussed this at the local and national level.

> Starting every Saturday, hundreds of leaders from the provincial level, the private sector and civil society met in the President's office. This went on for a whole year. Five major problems emerged from these discussions at the local and national level:

> 1.   Ensuring security
> 2.   Establishing unity in the country.
> 3.   Developing programs for justice and reconciliation
> 4.   Establishing good governance and democracy
> 5.   Rebuilding the economy[22]

At the local level these discussions used the traditional process called Ubudehe. It is a participatory process developed from a traditional practice of working collectively in agriculture. Ubudehe took place when all social and ethnic groups prepared the fields for the planting season. These forums also became the foundation for the constitutional discussion, preparing the country's first request for assistance from the international donor community, and later once the decentralisation process was implemented, became a process for budgeting and planning at the village level, where citizens allocate decentralized funds according to village priorities.[23]

This process was also used to elicit citizen's views on using Gacaca to deal with the genocide perpetrators. In 1999 as the country began to organize for the Gacaca process, a team from Johns Hopkins University working with the Center for Conflict Management at the National University of Rwanda (NUR) developed a household survey that was conducted between September and October 2000. Over 1600 people (1676) were interviewed in five provinces. Prisoners were included in the survey. The findings of their surveys were remarkably close to the initial discussions organized by Minister Musoni in 1999 in that issues related to poverty and safety were the highest concerns.[24]

The five priorities that emerged from the Ubudehe process were used as the basis for an Interim Poverty Reduction Strategy Paper (PRSP) that was submitted to the International Monetary Fund and World Bank in 1997. The PRPS formed the basis for assistance as well as debt relief and is a key document that structures major donor's assistance. The geno-cidal government of President Habyarimana had borrowed millions from the IMF and World Bank and Rwanda's new leaders were expected to repay the entire amount.

The participatory process of preparing the PRSP at the local level was used deliberately by Rwanda's new leaders to help reduce insecurity and conflict. The Ubudehe discussions continued for close to two years. The World Bank concluded of Rwanda's early efforts:

> The Rwanda PRS implementation process was reinforced by a well-structured approach to consultations; which were consciously used to include war-affected groups and prevent further violence. . . . Conflict mitigation mechanisms were incorporated into cellule-level consultations (cellule was the lowest level of administration in Rwanda containing about 200 households), which linked participatory rural appraisal methodologies (PRA) with the traditional concept of ubudehe in order to root participation in traditional processes. . . . In Rwanda citizens had rarely been involved in decision-making and social exclusion was one factor underlying the conflict. The authorities demonstrated a firm political commitment to consultative processes; consultations were consciously used to prevent further outbreaks of violence; and participatory processes included war-affected groups. . . . Further engagement with citizens was institutionalized as a tool for enriching political processes.[25]

While discussions continued weekly, at the local level in Ubudehe, the Saturday meetings at the President's office led to the formulation of a powerful and far-reaching vision for the country. The participants in Village Urugwiro were honest about the legacy of genocide, the poverty of the country, and the immense challenges facing leaders and citizens alike. The only way out of poverty and conflict, they included was to grow the economy, make sure the poor benefited, and include everyone in the process of decision-making. It sounded impossible, but they had few choices.

The questions posed in Village Urugwiro were the most basic: How do Rwandans envisage their future? What kind of society do they want to become? How can they construct a united and inclusive Rwandan identity? What are the transformations needed to emerge from a deeply unsatisfactory social and economic situation? These are the main questions Rwanda Vision 2020 addresses.

The forward of the first draft, written by Donald Kaberuka then the Minister for Finance and Economic Planning captures the spirit and focus of this vision and strategic plan. It is quoted at length because it forms the basis for the country's approach to good governance, human development, economic growth, the role of information technology, and the importance of ensuring gender equity and widespread access to education and health. As such, it can be considered one of the founding documents for post-genocide Rwanda.

> In 1998-1999, the Office of the President of the Republic of Rwanda launched national reflection sessions on the future of Rwanda in Village Urugwiro. After successful efforts in breaking the cycle of violence that had blighted Rwanda for 50 years, culminating in the horrifying genocide, the Government of National Unity felt the time had come for us, Rwandans to start thinking about what kind of Nation we want in the future.

> After extensive consultations, the Government of National Unity drafted a document called VISION 2020. This draft document was presented to a large cross-section of Rwandan society, by whom it was amended and validated. The final result is the current document, in which a long-term development path for Rwanda is outlined and ambitious goals to be reached by the year 2020 are formulated.

> VISION 2020 is a framework for Rwanda's development, presenting the key priorities and providing Rwandans with a guiding tool for the future. It supports a clear Rwandan identity, whilst showing ambition and imagination in overcoming poverty and division. The Rwandan Government, together with its partners, donors, civil society organisations and the private sector, is now in the process of formulating more detailed sectoral plans in order to attain the goals of VISION 2020.

> . . . Rwanda is one of the poorest countries in the world and we, the people of Rwanda, were until recently, and strongly divided. Hence,

VISION 2020 expresses the aim of attaining per capita income of a middle-income country in an equitable way, and the aspiration to become a modern, strong and united nation, without discrimination between its citizens. We identified six priority pillars and three cross-cutting areas, the development of which will be crucial for making the necessary long term transformations in Rwandan society happen and thus attaining the goals outlined above. The crucial task ahead of us is to make these key pillars and cross-cutting areas move in tandem. They touch upon most aspects of Rwandan society, and comprise socio-political and economic issues. . . .

Good governance is the topic of the first pillar, which affects a lot of spheres of Rwandan life and success in which will be crucial in fulfilling the promises of the VISION 2020. The other five pillars are mainly to do with economic development in a broad sense and are interdependent. It is outside the purpose of VISION 2020 to come up with details on strategies and policies, but it may be clear that we will always have to build upon our agricultural sector and develop it into productive and market-oriented agriculture over the medium term. . . .

At the core of our development process will be what constitutes Rwanda's principal asset: its people. Human resources will be improved, so that Rwanda can become a knowledge-based economy. In particular, we will actively encourage science and technology education and ICT skills, which will also help in addressing the fact that our country is landlocked. Whilst another cross-cutting areas; gender equality and environmental and natural resource management, are goals to be pursued in their own right, they will also contribute to the development of the other pillars and the overall goals of the VISION. . . .

Success in the implementation of VISION 2020 will depend primarily on the efforts and sacrifices of ourselves, the citizens of Rwanda. . . . Vision 2020 is to be achieved in a spirit of social cohesion and equity, underpinned by a capable state. However, we also agree that the current needs of Rwanda are enormous and that these will continue to be so, even within the VISION 2020 horizon. As such, whilst we will not shy away from our own responsibilities and reducing aid dependency substantially is a key component of Vision 2020, it is clear that donor support will remain necessary to successfully attain the goals outlined in this document.

Economic growth, alone, is not sufficient to bring about the necessary rise in the standard of living of the population. To vanquish hunger and poverty, growth must be Pro-Poor; giving all Rwandan's the chance to gain from the new economic opportunities. Vision 2020 aspires for Rwanda to become a modern, strong and united nation, proud of its fundamental values, politically stable and without discrimination amongst its citizens.[26]

Building Democracy:
Phase One of Decentralization

While Ubudehe was under way, the first national conference on governance was held in January 1998, and an Interim Governance Program (1998-2000) developed. The resulting plans for governance established goals and principles for good governance both at the national and local level, but the decentralization process was to lead the way in poverty reduction, delivery of services, accountability and direct democracy. The Ministry of Local Government and Social affairs was created in 1999-2000 and quickly generated the first Decentralisation Policy. It was drafted in 1999, and approved in 2000. It enshrines the goals and principles of decentralization and a proposed devolution of power. "The GOR recognizes that devolution of power, authority and resources plays a vital role on the fight against poverty. Through its policy of decentralisation people at the grass-root will be empowered to identify their needs and seek their satisfaction under the leadership of elected local authorities."[27]

Based on the original surveys that began at the end of the genocide, the decentralisation process was seen as a conflict mitigation mechanism, a way to build democratic participation, as well as a way over time to deliver services to the poor. The objectives of this program were laid out in the preface to the National Decentralisation Policy:

- To enable and reactivate, local people's participation, in initiating, making, implementing and monitoring decisions and plans that concern them
- To strengthen accountability and transparency in Rwanda by making local leaders directly accountable to the communities
- To enhance the sensitivity and responsiveness of public administration to the local environment by placing the planning, financing, management and control of service provision at the point where services are provided

- To develop sustainable capacity for economic planning and management at all levels
- To enhance effectiveness and efficiency in the planning, monitoring and delivery of services[28]

The principle of active, inclusive participation, with local communities defining their needs along with strategies for solving problems, combined with regular monitoring and evaluation are all part of this citizen-based governance model. The elements were established in the early post-genocide years and have become more embedded over time at the local and national level.

The first phase of decentralization, from 2000-03, concentrated on building the legal and administrative framework for decentralized governance, holding the first elections at the village level in 2000, and training both newly elected leaders as well as other members of the population about the new laws and responsibilities.

At the same time, during this first phase, fiscal decentralization began with the establishment of the Common Development Fund (CDF) that channels resources from the central government to local government. Initially only 1% of domestic revenue was transferred for local governments' activities but in 2003 this was increased to 3%. Over time the CDF and the process of decentralization began to gain the confidence of donors, especially the European Community who remain large contributors to decentralization.

An early evaluation of the decentralization process funded by the EU found the following:

- *Districts have been preparing regularly their annual budgets and projects proposals for submission to CDF.* The relation between resources and responsibilities of districts has been closely monitored leading to territorial and administrative reforms in 2005 aimed towards improving the fiscal capacities of districts and bringing services closer to the people through further devolution of responsibilities to the sector level and by reinforcing capacities at district level.
- *Fiscal transfers have been introduced to match the increase in district responsibilities. Modalities for the Community Development Fund (CDF) are now operational.* CDF was established to facilitate and monitor the flow of funds and

management information between the centre and the districts. Development budget transfers through CDF have increased on an annual basis from 2.7 billion RWF in 2003/2004 to 8.4 billion in 2005, indicating a gradual increase towards meeting the 10% target for development transfer. Since the year 2003, 3 percent of total domestic revenue is being transferred to support recurrent expenditure of the local governments.

Fiscal transfers to districts, also through the CDF, have been lower than anticipated, due to limited planning and absorption capacities of the districts. The transfer of resources has not matched the political transfer of responsibilities but local government's own revenue raising could be significantly strengthened. But service delivery, especially to the poor did not improve substantially nor was poverty significantly reduced.[29]

The slow progress in reducing poverty led the Minister of Local Governance, Protais Musoni, to conclude that more radical and fundamental changes needed to be made. It was determined that poverty could not be reduced faster without greater participation by the poor. Ubudehe and Imihigo were reborn.

Consolidation: 2003-2008

Security

The fundamental priority for Rwanda, especially in the transition period from 1994-2003 was to establish peace and security. Rwanda has made remarkable progress since 1994 in ensuring safety and security within its borders. There are several international and regional measures that bear this out.

The Global Peace Index, a ranking of countries on peace and security both within a country's borders as well as its level of militarization, places Rwanda 76 out of 140 countries on this index of peace and security. Developed by the Economist Intelligence Unit, the ranking includes measures of education, material well-being, and levels of democracy and transparency. Rwanda places ahead of many countries in the region as well as other much larger developing countries like India, Thailand and the Philippines. The measures include the number of homicides per 100,000 (an indicator where Rwanda scores among the best) and military expenditures as a percentage of GDP, again a measure where Rwanda shows very positive improvement in reducing this expenditure.[30]

The 2008 Mo Ibrahim Safety and Security Index, also a global ranking, places Rwanda very favorably in the East African region. An additional indicator of security within the country is that millions of refugees have returned. Between 1994 and 2002, 3,261,218 refugees returned to Rwanda: 16% from Burundi, 26.9% from Uganda, 10.2% from Uganda 46.2 from the Democratic Republic of the Congo.[31]

Military expenditures have declined significantly since 1998, and the Rwandan army, considered one of the most disciplined and effective on the continent, has downsized by 40,000 soldiers. Currently Rwanda has 3,000 peacekeepers in Sudan. Serious challenges continue with the Ex-FAR Interhamwe and FDLR, the perpetrators of the genocide, continuing to operate from Eastern Congo. Rwanda removed its troops from Congo in fall, 2002 as a UN Observation Mission in Congo (MONUC) was installed that took small steps toward disarming the Interhamwe and ex-FAR. From 2002 until late 2008 this region was relatively stable and secure with serious fighting erupting again in August 2008.

Figure 3.1
Poverty and Reductions in Military Expenditures

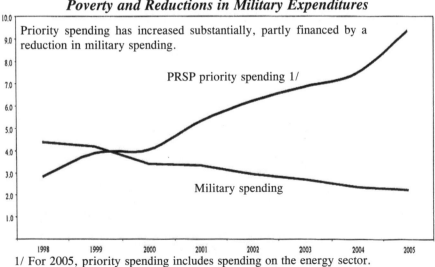

Priority spending has increased substantially, partly financed by a reduction in military spending.

PRSP priority spending 1/

Military spending

1/ For 2005, priority spending includes spending on the energy sector.

Source: *Rwanda: Fifth Review Under the Three Year Arrangement: Poverty Reduction and Growth Facility*, IMF, September 2005, p. 18.

Accountability

Based on the conceptual framework outline in chapter two, the key questions to address with regard to freedom, democracy and participation are:

- Are citizens involved in decision making about issues they value and
- Has the country made progress in establishing democracy?

Specifically, has Rwanda made progress in developing decision-making structures that are inclusive and that allow everyone to participate regardless of ethnic background and make choices about what they value.

During the transition period, from 1994-2003, establishing security and building consensus among parties and leaders was more of a priority that developing a multi-party model of democracy. Much of that changed with the constitution being implemented in 2003, and with the removal of restrictions on multiparty campaigning at the local level in 2007.

The Constitution

A country's constitution sets the framework not only for the philosophy of governing, but the political structures and processes that are allowed and forbidden. In 1999 a Constitution and Judicial Commission (CJC) was established to collect the views of the population on a Constitution and to prepare a draft constitution. It is widely acknowledged that this process was highly participatory. Meetings continued with the local population to obtain their views on what should be included in the Constitution. The most important accomplishment in establishing the rule of law, respect for human rights, commitment to democracy and gender equity is Rwanda's Constitution.

> The constitution commission was charged with the responsibility of collecting information. Questionnaires were distributed to the general population—every institution gave opinions on what it should be. The Commission collected these and then a team of experts drafted it. The drafting took 2-3 years. Then there were more discussions. The draft was distributed. There were many seminars. In 2003 the constitution passed.[32]

The constitutional committee finished their work in early 2002 and it was put to the voters. It was approved by 93% of those voting (with 87% of registered voters participating) in May 2002, and officially adopted on June 4th 2003 in a national referendum. It enshrines the fundamental rights of all citizens' and the country's approach to governance and equity. It establishes the principle of multiparty democracy, respect for human rights and gender equity, outlaws all forms of discrimination, including ethnic discrimination (Article 11) and sets as a goal, "the eradication of ethnic, regional and other divisions, and promotion of national unity."

The separation of powers was institutionalized. The judiciary became independent of the executive and legislative branch. Two chambers of Parliament were established. The Office of Ombudsman and Office of Auditor General were established to fight corruption. Gender equity was enshrined with the requirement that 30% of government positions be held by women. An annual meeting (Umushyikirano) between the President, Parliament, Judiciary and local government officials was also included. The dialogue that began in 1994 became enshrined in the new Constitution.

Legislature

On October 10, 2003 the new Members of a bicameral Parliament were sworn in. The 80 members of Parliament and 20 Senators were elected not appointed. In the first few weeks they exerted their independence by arguing successfully for a budget increase for their operations, investigated Gacaca-related killings, and sent a bill back to the executive branch for reconsideration on land expropriations. For the first time the Members of Parliament opened their committee meetings to the public, something that had not happened during the transition period, and which indicated a shift toward more transparency. Of the 80 members of Parliament, 53 are elected on a party basis using proportional representation, 24 seats are allocated to women, 2 for youth and 1 for the disabled.

Several human rights organizations state that there is no separation of powers in Rwanda, that the executive branch controls the legislature and the judiciary. After the publication of the favorable Mo Ibrahim Safety and Security index, Human Rights Watch claimed: "Neither the legislative nor the judiciary branches are independent of the RPF party or provide oversight of the executive." In fact, there are several provisions in the constitution that ensure separation of powers among parties. Article 116 says that no more than half of the positions in the Cabinet may be held by the political party gaining the majority of seats in the Chamber of Deputies. Secondly the President and Speaker of the Chamber must belong to different political parties (Article 58).

An independent evaluation conducted by the joint staffs of the World Bank and the International Monetary Fund that evaluated the first poverty reduction strategy concluded the following:

> The progress report points to significant progress in the area of political and economic governance. A new constitution was approved by referendum in May 2003 and a comprehensive review of legislation is in process . . . the progress report indicates that decentralization is advancing well.[33]

Elections

Rwanda has held both local and national elections since the genocide. The first elections were held at the local level for cell and sector councils five years after the genocide, in 1999. These elections were the first step in implementing this vision and program of decentralization. These were done by the queuing system where people who are running for office form a line and supporters line up behind their candidate of choice, not by secret ballot. The government asserted that this method was cheaper and simpler. Many organizations claimed that it initially allowed for continuing political control.

The second elections were held in 2000 when the Transitional National Assembly elected then Major-General Paul Kagame as President on April 22, 2000. Later in that year, in October 2000, Parliament passed a far-reaching law replacing a centralized political structure with a decentralized one. This was the beginning of a process of devolution of power authority and resources from the center to the local level that has allowed new and innovative local democratic processes to emerge.

District level elections followed in October 2000 and in February 2001 with new district level structures. In March 2001, Rwanda announced and established a new institution dedicated to running and monitoring the election process, the National Election Commission. In August 2003, Rwandan held its first post-genocide presidential election. It was also the first since independence that involved more than one party. While there were numerous complaints and reports from human rights and election monitoring organizations that the process was not transparent and free from interference, most agreed that Paul Kagame had won the election, if not at the reported rate of 96%.

For the 2003 elections, political parties were required to participate in a Forum of Political Organizations. This requirement has led some to conclude that the political parties have far less freedom than in other newly emerging democracies. But, in 2007, most restrictions on parties (except those involved in the genocide) had been removed and campaigning was allowed at all levels for local elections that were held in September 2008.

Justice

What we came up with was neither a civil law system, nor common law. It was a hybrid that we thought would work for Rwanda. Now people from other countries, Uganda, and Kenya are coming to look at our system. At the end of 2002 we had submitted to Cabinet for transmission to Parliament over 13 drafts dealing with criminal law and procedure, civil procedure, evidence, the organization and competence of courts, the establishment of the Supreme Court, the prosecution service, and the national prosecutor's office. It has all changed. If the court has decided then it is final. One of things we tried to achieve is independence of (the) judiciary from (the) political structure, from the executive. We did. The executive branch does not have a say.[34]

Trust and legitimacy cannot exist in a country without an independent judiciary and impartiality in dispensing justice. After a five-year review, discussion and analysis the Justice Sector Reform was completed in 2004. It is a far-reaching reform. It included, as Judge Busingye indicates, the creation of new institutions as well as the reform of existing ones. The reforms led to the enactment of new courts, procedures, academic and professional standards, and administrative and regulatory frameworks. An IMF review of the country's poverty reduction strategy concluded the following about the justice sector:

Major progress was achieved in governance over the PRSP period, with constitutional reform, national presidential and legislative elections in 2003, local elections in 2006, roll-out of *gacaca* community courts, improved relations with the international community and neighboring countries, and significant reductions in reported crime. Several reforms were undertaken in public, corporate and civic sectors by introducing new laws and new governance institutions while revamping old ones to ensure effective service delivery, better financial management, democratic governance, and low corruption. . . . The new constitution has provided a framework for representation and participation of citizens, bringing into existence key institutions including the two chambers of Parliament, an independent judiciary, the Prosecutor General's Office, the National Electoral Commission, the Office of the Ombudsman and the Office of the Auditor-General, among others.[35]

For the first time in the country's history, the reforms established an independent and decentralized prosecutor's office and educational standards. All judicial and prosecution officers now need a first degree in law, which has resulted in a significant improvement in the effectiveness of the justice sector staff. These reforms also led to the establishment of an Institute of Legal Practice and Development (ILDP), which is a permanent program for training judges and prosecutors, as one of the most pressing issues is the need for judicial education and training. Judicial reforms also included a new process for conflict resolution and mediation. In addition to establishing the Gacaca courts the new laws established mediation committees, also known as Abunzi, which are intended to encourage the settlement of disputes at the local level. Now mediation must occur before litigation in the courts. Over fifteen hundred Abunzi Mediation committees have been established for dispute resolution, and are focused especially on land disputes. In addition to reducing the caseload in courts, Abunzi has provided a cheap and easier process of obtaining legal remedies for the general population by bringing justice closer to the people. All mediators received training in conflict management. Consequently, instead of fines and other punishments previously used conflict management techniques are used in the mediation process.

The process of judicial reform that Judge Busingye discussed is far reaching. Rwanda has established an independent judiciary, modernized laws, and is working to complete the Gacaca trials. A large backlog of cases and improving legal education and training for judges and expanding the financial resources necessary for investigations and judicial processes are some of the most prominent challenges. Increasing access to the judicial system for the poor is also an important priority.

Gacaca

A pilot phase for this transitional form of justice, based on a traditional method of conflict resolution where trials are held outside in the "grass" (Gacaca is the Kinyarwanda word for grass) ran from 2005-2006 with 7,015 trials completed.[36] During this phase the number of suspects grew exponentially from 100,000 to over a million, mainly due to the process of Gacaca where suspects are encouraged to confess their crimes and name any other accomplices. By 2006 there were over 12,000 Gacaca courts with 170,000 judges. Over a million cases had been heard by the end of 2007.

Table 3.2
Completed Gacaca Trials 2006-2008

Level	Number of Trials	Pronounced Judgments	Remaining Case
Cell Level Category 3 only	612,151	557,607	54,554 (9%)
Sector Level	444,455	434,827	9,628 (2.1%)
Appeal Level	71,100	66,864	4,236 (5.9%)
TOTAL	1,127,706	1,059,298	68,408 (6%)

Source: National Service of Genocide Courts. *The Gacaca Courts Process: Implementation and Achievements*, February 2008.

While the judges received some legal training, the process has been criticized by some human rights organizations as not meeting Western legal standards as suspects are not given individual legal defense. In fact as Gacaca trials were being organized, I waited outside the office of the then Deputy-Prosecutor General Martin Ngoga as a regional representative for Amnesty International was leaving. "These trials are not fair—there is no legal representation for the defendants and judges have little training," said the Amnesty representative in a loud voice. "Send us lawyers," Ngoga replied, "Because otherwise what is the alternative?"

Gacaca has had far reaching implications. As of mid-2009 1,127,706 trials have been completed, about 94% of the total cases. Research into its effectiveness in providing reconciliation and justice is on going.[37] A Joint Governance Assessment published in October 2008 concluded, "The

Gacaca system is widely perceived as a step towards national reconciliation and appears to command popular legitimacy despite recognition of
its shortcomings. In view of the overwhelming caseload, there was probably no viable alternative, and Rwanda deserves much credit for addressing a daunting challenge in an impressive, ordered and consensual
manner."[38] For some of the survivors, Gacaca has not been an adequate
response to the murder of family members. Especially in the early years,
survivors, witnesses and judges were threatened and some killed. Even
with all of these problems a survey of public perceptions conducted by
the National University of Rwanda, with assistance from an international
organization, found the following: 95% of survivors and 80% of detain-
ees viewed the Gacaca system as more efficient than the ordinary courses.
81% of victims and 48% of defendants had confidence in the integrity of
the judges. The greatest problem identified was the high level of fear and
insecurity experienced by the judges (67%) victims (93%) and defendants (61%).[39] In contrast to Gacaca, the International Criminal Tribunal for Rwanda (ICTR) that was established by the United Nations to
deal with the organizers of the genocide has heard only 45 cases (39
convictions and 6 acquittals) at the cost of several billion dollars. Both
Gacaca and the ICTR are scheduled to complete their work by 2010.

Rwanda's educational system is not shying away from discussing the
genocide and the Gacaca method used to deal with the perpetrators. A
Macmillan primary six social studies text used throughout the country
has this powerful assignment:

Figure 3.2
Grade 6 Assignment on Genocide

> Write down the terms *genocide* and *massacre*.
> Explain what each term means. What reasons do
> you think one group might have for wanting to
> injure or destroy another group in this way?

> Why do you think the government
> called the Tuti insurgents inyenzi?

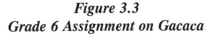

Figure 3.3
Grade 6 Assignment on Gacaca

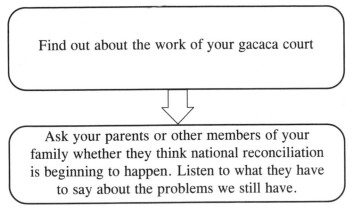

In 2007, one of the authors set an appointment to re-interview Tharcisse Karugarama who then was Minister of Justice and Attorney General. We waited patiently outside his office while a stream of people entered. When finally he asked us to come in he said: "What kind of legal problems are you having?" I was a bit stunned and explained the purpose of my interview. "Oh, today is the day anyone in the country can come to see me with their problems and complaints."

A joint governance assessment conducted by Rwanda's major donors concluded the following in 2008:

Rwanda had no real experience of a professional and independent judiciary prior to 1994. Furthermore, what did exist was virtually destroyed during the genocide when many judges and lawyers were murdered and others fled the country. Legal capacity had to be totally rebuilt at the same time as the country has had to deal with massive numbers of genocide suspects awaiting trial. In 2000-1 Rwanda began a programme of major judicial reform aiming to strengthen the independence of the judiciary, to improve the professionalism of the system, to reduce the case backlog and to ensure that judges and lawyers are appropriately qualified. The most important measures included the introduction of single-judge trials at lower levels (all trials had previously required three judges), minimum qualifications for judges, strict rules on *habeas corpus* (a 30 day limit on detention before charge), legal limitations on time period for delivering judgements (6 months after judges receive files), ending of the role of the Ministry of Justice in budgetary and recruitment decisions, creation of independent budgets for the Office of the Public Prosecutor and Supreme Court, and the creation of an independent Inspectorate General. At the same time as these reforms have taken place Rwanda has modernised its framework of laws, including a major revision to the Penal Code in 2004. Rwanda has progressively developed human resource capacity in the legal sector. The Rwandan Bar Association, which was established in 1997, now has 273 members, 54 of whom are women. The reforms in the legal sector have strengthened the formal independence of the judiciary and improved its quality.[40]

Corruption

One of the major reforms involves the creation of the Auditor General's Office (OAG) in 1999 to audit government adherence to fiscal controls and the Office of the Ombudsman 2004 to investigate and fight public and private corruption. It is an independent office that investigates and prosecutes corruption. The Ombudsman's office has been very aggressive at identifying corruption and has also developed a corruption ranking for government institutions. Reducing corruption has been a high priority of the Rwandan government and it has paid off. The World Bank's governance measures show that Rwanda has made significant progress in controlling corruption, ranking among the highest in the region with Botswana and Mauritius.[41] Corruption flourishes where civil and political rights are absent. Conversely as a country improves its record on political and civil rights, and allows for increasing freedom, corruption is reduced. This is a large part of what is occurring in Rwanda.

Freedom of the Press

In pre-genocide Rwanda, the press, Kangura and radio station, RTLM were deeply involved in both inciting the hate that led to the genocide as well as participating in the genocide through announcing where people were hiding. Radio-Television Libres des Milles Collines (RTLM) was the voice of Hutu Ideology.[42]

On December 3, 2003 the ICTR convicted the directors of RTLM, Ferdinand Nahimana and Jean-Bosco Barayagwiza of genocide, incitement to commit genocide and crimes against humanity.

Because of the media's involvement in the genocide, the press until recently has been regulated, with serious restrictions on sectarianism and promoting genocide ideology. A 2001 law, On The Prevention, Suppression and Punishment of the Crime of Discrimination and Sectarianism makes it a crime to promote hate speech. One of the challenges with the law is its vagueness and determining whether individuals have the intent to commit hate speech. The law is being rewritten, and the challenge is to balance the need to ensure that genocide ideologies are not given a voice with freedom to report. However, levels of security and education have improved to such an extent in the country and the Government of Rwanda has recently expanded the space for freedom of expression. It is fair to now say that the press has broad freedoms in Rwanda.

Every year, the International Research and Exchange Board (IREX) an NGO supported in part by USAID, conducts an annual survey "of the conditions for independent media." Called the Media Sustainability Index (MSI), in 2007, for the first time, it included African countries in its analysis. MSI assesses five objectives related to freedom of the press:

1. Legal and social norms present to protect and promote free speech and access to public information
2. Whether journalism meets professional standards of quality
3. Whether multiple news sources exist to prove citizens with reliable and objective news
4. Whether independent media are well-managed businesses. Allowing editorial independence and
5. Whether supporting institutions function in the professional interests of independent media[43]

According to IREX, "the scoring is done in two parts. First a panel of experts is assembled in each country, drawn from representatives of local media, NGOs, professional associations, international donors, and media-development implementers. . . . The panelists scores are reviewed by IREX in-country staff and Washington D.C., media staff, which then score the countries independently of the MSI panel. Using the combination of scores, the final scores are determined."[44] All countries scores are tabulated and then an average for the region is attained, Averages for all countries reviewed in Africa (37 countries) from best scores to worst are: Objective 5 supporting institutions (2.20); Objective 3, plurality of news (2.04); Objective 1, free speech (1.94); Objective 2, professional journalism (1.81) and Objective 4, business management (1.63).[45]

On the MSI, Rwanda received an overall score of 2.9, which according to IREX "reflects fairly strong scores in Objectives 1 and 3, freedom of speech and plurality of news. On the lower end, Objectives 4 and 5, business management and supporting institutions, scored just above and just below 2, respectively." IREX's Rwanda Report recommends numerous changes that are needed in Rwanda including increasing the professionalism and pay for journalists, and removing Press Law 2002 that restricts access to some public information and Cabinet minutes. The Report, conducted by the East African Journalist Association also includes the following statements: "Licensing of both broadcast and print media is fair and very transparent. Anyone who wishes to start a radio and television station or newspaper is free to apply for a license and that it takes only a few days to be approved. There is no restriction on accessing foreign news sources by media outlets and the Internet can be used freely by those who can afford it (typically in urban areas) Some media depend on international news agencies and the Internet as their primary sources of international news, and they are free to publish or air this information in a language of their choice."[46]

It is worth reflecting on this independent analysis of Rwanda's media because one of the primary criticisms of human rights organizations is that there are no press freedoms in Rwanda, that it is a one-party state with little or no freedom for the press. On April 2008, the Executive Director of the Human Rights Watch wrote in an op-ed in the *Los Angeles Times*:

> Rwanda has a long way to go. Despite the façade of occasional elections, the government essential runs a one-party state. Under the guise of preventing genocide, the government displays a marked intolerance of the most basic forms of dissent. There is no meaningful opposition. The press is cowed.[47]

It is impossible to reconcile the picture of Rwanda presented by Human Rights Watch and objective, independent analytical studies that have been conducted on press freedoms, and it is worth asking: what is the basis for their views? What is the evidence that "the press are cowed" in Rwanda." Who holds Human Rights Watch accountable for their views?

In reading and translating the local papers one sees an even greater plurality of opinions. There are 62 newspapers in Rwanda (with 15 active) 51 registered print outlets, 16 radio stations. The majority are in Kinyarwanda. A careful examination of local newspapers and radio shows conducted in Kinyarwanda shows a high level of freedom of speech, debate and criticism of the government. Important national and local issues are debated fiercely; leaders are criticized and policies evaluated.

In fact, the majority of the population receives its information through radio, not the press. Recently, numerous "call-in" radio stations have been launched. Tom Ndahiro, the former human rights commissioner and scholar, is the host of one of those radio shows. "I interview whoever I want and ask any questions. I have interviewed the President three times in two years," he said in November 2008.

Local Governance and Decentralization: Ubudehe and Imihigo

Remarkable and unique changes in political structures and authority have occurred at the local level. In only fifteen years, central control has evolved into devolution of power and resources to the lowest levels. Exclusion has become inclusion; voices are heard from the weakest, poorest and most vulnerable. It is far from perfect but it is building a culture of democracy and accountability.

"Today we are reviewing the District's draft plans for 2006. Each Mayor has ten minutes to make their presentations, and then we will hear comments." After the introduction by the Minister of Primary Education, the mayors from each of the districts began presenting power points listing goals for their districts. One of the primary goals for all of the districts was "modern latrines" for the schools. At the end of all the presentations the Prime Minister, Bernard Makuza stood up. He said, "It is not acceptable that our children do not have modern latrines. I will find the money from my budget to ensure that all schools have modern latrines by the time schools starts in 6 weeks."

What had I witnessed? What were the PowerPoint's of goals and objectives? Why were most of the senior leaders of the country reviewing these plans, making comments? I had witnessed the rebirth of processes called Ubudehe and Imihigo.

Imihigo was a traditional ritual that occurred when a group of people came together and engaged publicly in activities that tested their bravery. The community, as well as the individual was being tested. Now Imihigo means something quite different. It is a public declaration of what is valued and needed by individuals and communities and a commitment to achieve a specified set of goals.

The process of determining community needs is called Ubudehe. It starts with each family and moves up to the level of 100 families—called umudugudu—then through the cell, sector and district level where these needs and commitments become a contract (Imihigo) that is signed by the Mayor of each district and the President. The contract includes a set of measurable performance indicators for one year that the mayor is expected to achieve. The goals are set after extensive conversations with the local populations. District mayors engage their communities to understand what the needs are, how they relate to Vision 2020 and the Millennium Development Goals. Each Imihigo is unique but categorized in several areas: social protection, governance, health, education, economic development, agriculture, and justice.

In 2007 I visited Mayor John Vianney Murego in Gatsibo District, that is located along the Ugandan border, to see how the Ubudehe system works and to talk to him about his Imihigo. He explained how the system worked and then he talked to poor farmers and asked them what the government could do to solve their problems. With his community, Mayor Kabonero established targets in health, education and water access that he must meet each year or he will lose his job. His performance contract says:

I, Mayor John Vianney Murego, in the name of the population that I represent, I pledge to the President of the Republic that during the year 2006, the population of the District will achieve the objectives that are stated in this contract document. The Republic of Rwanda, through the ministries and other state institutions, is going to support the activity program described in the following document.

REPUBULIKA Y'U RWANDA

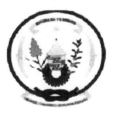

AMASEZERANO Y'IMIHIGO Y'AKARERE KA GATSIBO MU MWAKA WA 2007

Njyewe, **John Vianney MUREGO**, Umuyobozi w'Akarere ka GATSIBO, mw'izina ry'Abaturage nyobora, nemereye Nyakubahwa Perezida wa Repubulika y'u Rwanda, ko mu mwaka w'i 2007, Abaturage b'Akarere bazagera ku ntego zikubiye mu gitabo kiri ku mugereka w'aya masezerano.

Leta y'u Rwanda, ibinyujije muri za Minisiteri n'izindi nzego zirebwa na buri gikorwa, izadutera inkunga zinyuranye mu gushyira mu bikorwa iyo gahunda.

Bikorewe i Kigali, kuwa 20 Ukuboza 2006.

**Umuyobozi w'Akarere
Ka GATSIBO**

John Vianney MUREGO

**Perezida wa Repubulika
y'u Rwanda**

Paul KAGAME

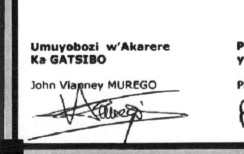

How does the community determine its needs? This is the process of Ubudehe.

First each family comes together and decides what resources they already have, what they need, and what they will commit to each other. These family needs (for example, a cow, money for schooling, food, employment) are then discussed at the level of the umudugudu when 100 families come together to discuss their collective and individual needs. Both the umudugu's resources as well as needs are mapped on a cloth using a social mapping process.

Figure 3.4
Social Mapping

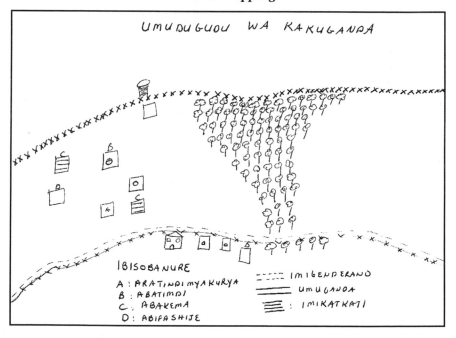

Individual dwellings are mapped along with their needs, as well as social categories such as widows, vulnerable children, and the absolute poor. Then eight people are chosen from the Umudugudu level to represent the collective needs. The Kakuganda umudugudu is represented in Figure 3.4. Once these eight are chosen they represent the Umudugudu at the level of the cell where two elected committees evaluate the Umudugudu plans. The committees, the Joint Action Development Forum (JADF) and the Community Development Committee (CDC) respectively, evaluate the plans and the resources needed to achieve the Ubudehe.

The result of these committees analysis is then passed to the level of the sector where each cell's plans are reviewed and evaluated. Members of both cell and sector committees are elected by secret ballot. Finally, the plans for all of the Umudugudu, cells and sectors reach the district. There can be up to 20 sectors in a district. At this point, the elected council reviews all of the plans and determines what will become part of the Imihigo for the community.

The council is also elected by secret ballot and can remove members—the Mayor and both Vice-Mayors for incompetence, failure to achieve the stated goals, and illegal or inappropriate behavior. In fact, since 2006, six mayors have been removed (two mayors in the Western Province two in the south, one in Kigali and one in the East) for incompetence and one for public drunkenness.

The executive committee, which consists of the Mayor and two Vice-mayors (one for economics and one social) is elected by an Electoral College formula where 1000 people in the district vote for the executive committee. The Electoral College is based on a formula to include youth, women, the disabled, and representatives from the sector, cell and umudugudu.

Ubudehe has grown from the first pilot with 600 cells in 2002 to more than 9154 cells in 2007. It has been funded jointly by the Government of Rwanda and the European Union. In 2008, Ubudehe won the prestigious United Nations Public Service Award. Over 150 countries participated and 12 programs were nominated.

According to the European Commission:

> A grassroots level development programme, jointly funded by the Government of Rwanda and the European Commission has been awarded the United Nations Public Service Award 2008. The prize recognises global excellence in public service in countries around the world. The Commission has financed the programme, known as the "Ubudehe" programme, since early 2001. So far a total of 25 million has been contributed for fighting rural poverty and improving local governance in Rwanda.

> The United Nations Public Service Awards Programme is the most prestigious international recognition of excellence in public service. The Awards programme was established in 2003 to promote profes-

sionalism in the public sector around the world, recognising that democracy and successful governance are built on a competent civil service. 150 countries participated in the 2008 competition. Rwanda was
amongst the 12 countries that have been honoured with an award. The
'Ubudehe' programme empowers citizens at community level in Rwanda
to plan and implement poverty reduction projects. The programme
was found to have fostered citizens' participation in policymaking while
having improved transparency, accountability and responsiveness in
the public service.[48]

Ubudehe and the Imihigo contract are unique in several respects.
They are accountability mechanisms that go beyond voting for a candidate. The Ubudehe process is inclusive and empowering. It engages the
poor in planning and decision-making as well as being a method for
identifying local problems and developing local solutions, and building a
culture of participation and accountability.

Ubudehe includes both devolution of power and resources because
the 3% transfer to the Community Development Fund ensures that funds
are being decentralized to match the process.

Rwanda has also used Citizen Report Cards and Community Score
Cards to rate public service delivery for education and health care at the
local level.[49] Citizen Report Cards originated with civil society organizations in India in 1993 to monitor public services in Bangalore. They
are now used around the world in both developing and developed countries Community Score Cards are a newer invention, which also focus on
monitoring accountability and responsiveness of service providers. Two
pilots were conducted four districts in 2004 and 2005. Users were sur-
veyed on their satisfaction of the quantity and quality of services in education and health care, with important information emerging about female education (girls drop out of school to look for jobs or as a result of
becoming orphans.) The surveys also showed the need for equipment
ranging from basic items such as books to computers and lab equipment.
Critical problems related to the cost of education and health care also
were documented in these citizen-based surveys.

Performance-based democratic structures may seem redundant. In a
democracy, elections are supposed to be the accountability mechanism
for removing officials from office. Holding elected officials accountable
for specific outcomes may ensure that at least in Rwanda, democratic
officials do their best to keep their promises. Performance based management has spread though the private sector around the world and to

some local governments in the United States.[50] It offers much promise for developing countries and those interested in development should examine the process carefully. This could be a component in a new model for the "development state."

In 2008, a joint governance assessment conducted by the World Bank, the major international donors including UNDP, the African Development Bank, USAID, SIDA, CIDA, GTZ and the Belgian Technical Cooperation Agency, with input from the Government of Rwanda, concluded the following about Rwanda's progress in accountability and inclusiveness:

> Accountability is essential to ensure that government works in the interest of citizens. . . . Horizontal accountability refers to the checks and balances existing between different governmental bodies (for example between the legislature and executive) aimed an ensuring adequate scrutiny and preventing abuse of power. Vertical accountability operates in an upwards and downwards direction between different levels of government and between government and citizens. All these forms of accountability exist in Rwanda. . . .

> Over the past few years they have been strengthened in important ways, notably through the 2003 Constitution that upholds multiparty democracy and mandates numerous bodies charged with monitoring government performance. . . . Rwanda has made significant progress in promoting inclusive governance. Fundamental to this change has been the approach chosen by Rwanda to reject any form of ethnic labeling, discrimination and representation in politics and government.[51]

Rwanda has come a long way since the terrible events of 1994. Security has improved tremendously. The rule of law has been strengthened. Corruption is very low. The judiciary is far more independent and effective than at any time in the country's history and especially at the local levels, and people are participating in unique forms of democratic decision-making.

Many challenges remain: there is a great need for more education and training in almost all areas of government, but especially for the judiciary, the media, for civil society organizations, for Members of Parliament and for the electoral commissions. Reconciliation will continue to be a major issue—possibly for generations—and far more resources are needed to implement and monitor government programs.

In July, 2008, after a long car ride from Kigali to near the Congo border to celebrate the opening of a local market and to visit an accountability day presentation with Minister Protais Musoni and the European Union Ambassador, David Macrae, Ambassador Macrae said, "the decentralisation process has lead to direct democracy and is beginning to reduce poverty. We are very pleased with the results."[52]

Notes

1. Interviews with Minister Protais Musoni, 2005-2008.

2. Appendix One contains the names of all individuals who have been interviewed for this book during the last decade.

3. See Christian Scherrer, *Genocide and Crisis in Central Africa: Conflict Roots, Mass Violence and Regional War*. Westport: Praeger Publishers, 2002. As he says, the "money solved very few problems; all it did was keep a deadly threat alive." p. 145145 Clearly much of the decade long struggle between genocidiares in the Congo and the government and people of Rwanda can be traced to this period and the funding of the so-called refugees.

4. See Daniela Kroslak, *The French Betrayal of Rwanda*. Bloomington: Indiana University Press, 2008.

5. Carol Rittner, John K. Roth and Wendy Whitworth. *Genocide in Rwanda: Complicity of the Churches?* Newark, U.K.: Aegis Publishers, 2004.

6. Daniel Kaufmann, A. Kraay and M. Mastruzzi. *Governance Matters VII: Governance Indicators for 1996-2007*. Washington D.C.: The World Bank, 2008.

7. Denis Goulet, "Participation in Development: New Avenues." *World Development* Vol. 17 No. 2 (1989): 165.

8. Phil Clark and Zachary Kaufman, "Introduction and Background: After Genocide." In Phil Clark and Zachary Kaufman eds. *After Genocide: Transitional Justice, Post-Conflict Reconstruction and Reconciliation in Rwanda and Beyond*. New York: Columbia University Press, 2009. P. 6.

9. See for example, African Rights, *Rwanda: Death, Despair and Defiance*. London: African Rights, 1995.Des Forges, A. *Leave None to Tell the Story: Genocide in Rwanda*. New York: Human Rights Watch, 1999, Dallaire, R. Shake Hands with the Devil: The Failure of Humanity in Rwanda. Toronto: Random House Canada, 2003.

10. Most of the documentation that is available is from donor reports, especially USAID and IMF reports. For example see Teschner, Douglass. "Analysis of the Legislative Process at the Rwanda Transitional National Assembly."

USAID/ ARD/SUNY: Project d' Appui a L'Assemblee Nationale du Rwanda, September 19, 2002.

11. Many of the refugees were in fact genocidiares who fled to the Congo where for more than a decade they conducted cross border raids into Rwanda.

12. Statement by Tom Ndahiro, June 29, 2009. Mr. Ndahiro was located along the Zairian border during this initial.

13. Douglass Teschner. "Analysis of the Legislative Process at the Rwanda Transitional National Assembly." USAID/ ARD/SUNY: Project d' Appui a L'Assemblee Nationale du Rwanda, September 19, 2002, p. 10.

14. United Nations Resolution 999 S/RES/955 (8 November 1994), p. 1.

15. These laws were superscded by the constitution which passed in 2003.

16. Douglass Teschner. "Analysis of the Legislative Process at the Rwanda Transitional National Assembly." USAID/ ARD/SUNY: Project d' Appui a L'Assemblee Nationale du Rwanda, September 19, 2002, p. 10, P. 8.

17. Interviews with Judge Busingye, July 2004-08. Busingye Johnstone is currently the President of the High Court of Rwanda.

18. Schabas, William A. "Post Genocide Justice in Rwanda: A Spectrum of Options." In Phil Clark and Zachary Kaufman eds. *After Genocide: Transitional Justice, Post-Conflict Reconstruction and Reconciliation in Rwanda and Beyond*. New York: Columbia University Press, 2009, p. 217.

19. One of the originators off the idea, Tharcisse Karugarama, is now Minister of Justice and in an interview in 2003 talked about the difficulty national leaders faced in determining a method to deal with the scope of those involved in the genocide.

20. Much of the criticism was to charges that the RPA had committed retribution killings, then to Gacaca.

21. Interviews with Tom Ndahiro, 2006-08.

22. Interviews, Minister Protais Musoni July 2004, July 2005, July 2006 and July and November 2008.

23. The World Bank's report, *Toward a Conflict-Sensitive Poverty Reduction Strategy: Lessons from a Retrospective Analysis*. Report 32587, published in 2005 analyzed post conflict reconstruction in 9 countries with an analysis of conflict reduction and nation building in Rwanda's early post-genocide years.

24. Johns Hopkins Center for Communications Programs. *Perceptions about the Gacaca Law in Rwanda: Evidence from a Multi-Method Study*. Special Publication No. 19. Baltimore: Johns Hopkins University School of Public Health, Center for Communication Programs. April, 2001.

25. World Bank, *Toward a Conflict-Sensitive Poverty Reduction Strategy: Lessons from a Retrospective Analysis*. Report 32587, P. 9 and 52.

26. Republic of Rwanda, Ministry of Finance and Economic Planning. Rwanda Vision 2020, 2000.

27. Republic of Rwanda, Ministry of Local Government and Social Affairs. Community Development Policy, May, 2000, P. 20.

28. Republic of Rwanda, Ministry of Local Government and Social Affairs. National Decentralization Policy. May, 2000, Preface.

29. Republic of Rwanda, Ministry of Local Government and Social Affairs. National Decentralization Policy. May 2000 and Republic of Rwanda, Ministry of Local Government and Social Affairs. Implementation Strategy for National Decentralization Policy. May, 2000.

30. Global Peace Index, Executive Summary www.visionofhumanity.org.

31. The Ibrahim Index of Safety and Security considers seven indicators to create the national rankings: 1) Number of armed conflicts in which a government is involved in that year 2) Intensity of the violent conflicts in the country in that year 3) The number of deaths due to intentional attacks on civilians by governments or formally-organized armed groups 4) Refugees and asylum seekers originating from each country 5) Internally displaced persons (IDPs) 6) Ease of access to small arms and light weapons 7) Level of violent crime. For more information see: www.moibrahimfoundation.org.

32. Interview with Judge Busingye, July 2006.

33. International Monetary Fund. *Rwanda: Joint Staff Assessment of the Poverty Reduction Strategy Paper*. IMF Country Report No. 04/274. August 2004, pp. 5-6.

34. Interview with Judge Busingye, July, 2007.

35. International Monetary Fund, Rwanda: Poverty Reduction Strategy Paper, IMF Country Report No. 08/90 (March 2008): pp. 24-25.

36. National Service of Genocide Courts, *The Gacaca Courts Process*, February 2008, Table 1.

37. An excellent analysis of post-genocide justice issues can be found in After Genocide: Transitional Justice, Post-conflict Reconstruction and Reconciliation in Rwanda and Beyond, edited by Phil Clark and Zachary Kauffman, New York: Columbia University Press, 2009.

38. Rwanda Joint Governance Assessment Report, August 3, 2008, p. 25.

39. Social Cohesion in Rwanda: An Opinion Survey (2005-07), National Unity and Reconciliation Commission (NURC) Table 2.

40. Rwanda: Joint Governance Assessment, October 2008, p. 28. The assessment included: "the ambassadors of the USA, UK, Belgium, the Netherlands, Swiss, EU and Germany, including heads of development agencies namely; the World Bank, AfDB, UNDP, USAID, SIDA, CIDA, DFID, Belgium Technical Co-operation, and the GTZ was put in place. Government's representation on the committee included a representative of the office of the President, Ministers of Local Government, Finance and Planning, Information, Public Service, Interior, Justice and Commerce. Relevant institutions on the committee also included the Ombudsman's Office, the Auditor General's Office, NEPAD, Rwanda Human Rights Commission, the Forum for Political Parties,

RALGA, International NGO Network, Rwanda Civil Society Platform, Rwanda Governance Advisory Council and the Private Sector Federation. The Steering Committee, jointly chaired by the Minister of Local Government and the World Bank Country Manager, was set up to lead and manage the JGA process. The SC was supported by a Joint Technical Committee comprising representatives from Government and development partners. . . . An international firm—The Policy Practice from the United Kingdom—was recruited through an open competitive process to carry out the JGA." From the Preface to the Assessment.

41. Kaufmann, D., A. Kraay and M. Mastruzzi. *Governance Matters VII: Governance Indicators for 1996-2007.* Washington D.C.: The World Bank, 2008.

42. See Thompson, Allan, ed. *The Media and the Rwanda Genocide.* London: Pluto Press, 2007.

43. www.irex.org/msi/index.asp.

44. Media Sustainability Index Overview, www.irex.org/msi/index.asp.

45. Media Sustainability Index Overview, www.irex.org/msi/ African summary.

46. IREX, Media Sustainability Index: Rwanda 2008, P. 4.

47. Kenneth Roth, "The Power of Horror in Rwanda," *Los Angeles Times*, April 11, 2009 Opinion Section.

48. European Union *Document IP/08/1202.* Brussels 24 July 2008, p. 1.

49. See Organization for Social Science Research in Eastern and Southern Africa. (OSSRESA) *Rwanda: Citizen Report Cards and Community Score Cards.* OSSRESA, 2006.

50. Julnes, Patria de Lancer, Frances Stokes Berry, Maria Aristigueta, and Kaifeng Yang eds. *International Handbook of Practice-Based Performance Management.* London: Sage, 2008, and Holzer, Marc and Kathryn Kloby. "Helping Government Measure Up: Models of Citizen Driven Government Performance Measurement Initiatives." In *International Handbook of Practice-Based Performance Management.* London: Sage, 2008.

51. World Bank, Rwanda *Joint Governance Assessment Report.* World Bank Country Manager, Kigali Rwanda. August 3, 2008, pp. 17-18.

52. Interview with Ambassador David MacRae, July 2008.

Chapter Four

Basic Needs: Education, Gender Equity and Health Care

Education

I became someone. The education added value to my life. Now, I want to become an engineer and build our society.

Jane Uwere, Form 12

I completed primary school in Tanzania. When I came here I did not have a voice. I did not see myself as being capable of doing anything. FAWE has helped me to feel confident, strong and comfortable.

Florence Mutesi, graduate in biology and chemistry

Boys are given more value. I have been able to live with people who have my dreams. I want to write about Rwanda so more people will come and understand our dreams. I am on a scholarship. I come from a large family and my dad is dead. I never thought I would study math and physics. I want to become a mechanical engineer.

Aziza, Form 11

These girls attend an all-girls secondary school in Rwanda. They are required to study math, science, and use advanced computer technologies. They come from all over the country. Most are very poor. All of the students have had to pass rigorous merit-based tests to be allowed to enter FAWE. "We do not accept students because their mother or their father is important, or in the government. They have to pass the test to be admitted. A girl attending secondary and tertiary education was once only a dream in this country. FAWE has made helped many girls make those dreams come true," said Sarah Besaje, Headmistress of FAWE School.

The FAWE (Forum for African Women in Education) girl's school in Kigali, Rwanda, puts to rest any doubt that girls are not equally qualified to study math and science, or that poor children cannot succeed at the same intellectual levels as the children of the rich.[1] FAWE is a public school located in Kigali city. It was founded in 1999 in partnership with the Ministry of Education to promote girls education and has four goals:

1. Increase the number of school places for girls
2. Reduce the social and domestic problems that girls face
3. Provide a conducive learning environment especially in sciences and math and
4. Empower girls to demonstrate their academic capabilities when given the right environment and opportunities.

The school has innovative and strong programs in leadership as well as a focus on reducing domestic violence, a significant problem that remains in present day Rwanda. The school started with 160 students and had 700 by fall, 2008 from form one to form six (grades 7-12). The academic performance of many of its graduates is impressive. It is consistently ranked among the top performing schools in the country and in 2004 the top student in the country overall as well as in science and math came from FAWE. "We are demonstrating that a girl is as capable as a boy . . . and girls who are empowered are able to become leaders. We want to prove to the world that if we have well-trained teachers and good equipment, our girls can not only can help rebuild our country but be as successful as any children in the world," said Sarah Besaje.

The FAWE girl's school represents many the goals and the achievements of Rwanda's education policy. The academic program focuses almost exclusively on math and science as the country's policy and vision is that knowledge of these fields will lay the basis for economic growth and productivity. Vision 2020, the governing strategic vision, is based on the notion that developing an educated populace who understands science and is familiar with using information technologies will be the primary way Rwandans becomes a knowledge-based society.

FAWE also represents the government's commitment to gender equity and the belief that everyone—including poor girls—can become scientists. Education is also seen as a factor in reducing poverty and economic growth as well as building tolerance and reconciliation in the country. "Education . . . is a fundamental strategy in promoting future peace and reconciliation through the development of independent thinking, unprejudiced and non-sectarian attitudes, as well as a commitment to human rights."[2]

Education progress in Rwanda is impressive, particularly at the primary school level. The net primary enrollment rate increased from 74% in 2000 to 95% in 2006. Improvement has occurred both in urban as well as rural areas. One of the primary drivers of this progress was the removal of tuition and fees in 2003. In addition teacher-training programs had led to a 40% increase in qualified, licensed primary school teachers during this same period. This progress is sufficient to project that Rwanda is on track to achieve one of the millennium goals as well as a Vision 2020 goal—universal primary enrollment by 2015.[3] Both primary and secondary schools are increasingly using a common core curriculum focusing on math and science and the use of technology.

Gender equity or parity in primary school enrollment was achieved in 2000 and according to the Ministry of Education is now higher for girls, at 87% than for boys. "By 2005 Rwanda had achieved the Education for All Goal of eliminating gender disparities in primary education in terms of attendance. However girls are lagging behind boys in terms of completion rates and on exam scores. . . . The Education for All Goal also emphasizes the need not only for girls to be present in school, but also for attention to be paid to their needs in relation to teaching and learning practices, curricula and the safety of the school environment."[4]

Primary and Secondary School Challenges

The Government of Rwanda has recently announced a commitment to fund nine years of basic education. This major new policy, called Nine Years Basic Education (9YBE) was implemented in 764 schools in 2009. This fee free nine years of education is almost unprecedented in the developing world—and once fully implemented could have major development implications, especially related to population growth and economic development. However, because of rapid population growth, which is described in the section on gender below, attaining this goal will be difficult without significant external funding.

The progress in improving enrollment rates at primary school, and gender parity are very impressive accomplishments in a fifteen-year period. The vision of becoming a knowledge based and technologically driven country will not be attainable, however with low levels of enrollment at the secondary and tertiary level.[5] Currently only 10% of children continue on to secondary school and 4% to intuition of higher learning.

A self-evaluation conducted by the Ministry of Education in 2006 concluded:

> There is a clear recognition across the sector of providing quality basic education . . . in quantity in order to develop Rwanda's human resources, to generate employment and thus to reduce poverty. Access to education has improved at all levels of the system . . . but the costs of schooling are still too high for poor families, and the percentage of children who actually complete a full cycle of primary school is below the Sub-Saharan average.[6]

Developing comprehensive programs to train teachers, especially in science and math, acquiring textbooks for all children, expanding access to secondary and higher education are some of the large challenges that will be eased once Internet access is widespread.

Challenges in Higher Education

In the post-genocide environment the Rwandan leadership faced an unprecedented situation. They understood the critical importance of education but at the same time were faced with an almost complete lack of human resources necessary to make an educational system function.[7] Furthermore, there were virtually no older educators or professors with experience and training due to the genocide. This meant that the Government needed to act quickly and decisively to create or to recruit the critical mass of educated leaders committed to the importance of a first rate education system which would drive the future of the country. In response to this need the Kagame government took several actions.

First the Government identified and recruited talented and already educated members of the Diaspora who were Rwandan and in many cases those who were not Rwandan. Second the Government entered into an aggressive policy of seeking opportunities for Rwandans to study outside of the country to obtain needed post graduate qualifications. Both of our universities have been partners to this strategy, educating Rwandans at our universities as well as within the country, especially in law and public health. Rwanda's openness and encouragement of outside involvement went far to open the doors of the traditional education system to new and interesting inputs from around the world. The existence of a traditional and slow-to-change higher education system can be as much of a barrier as an aide to rapid development. In Rwanda the open and progressive leadership has moved higher education in a faster better direction than its neighbors.

The final policy decision that helped put the country on an entirely different footing for potential education issues was the adoption of English as an official third language of the country. Most senior public officials had come mostly from outside the country, educated in other African countries (Uganda, Kenya, DROC) or in France, Belgium, the United Kingdom and the United States. Driven by the fact that the second language of many of the new leaders was English not French and by a desire to distance themselves from the French African Policy and educational system, the Government made the declaration that schooling was acceptable at all levels, if offered in English. This single decision opened the door for having teachers and professors from nearby Anglophone countries come and immediately integrate into the educational system as well as moving towards further and better relations in the East African Economic Community, most of which is Anglophone. It also aligned the country with the primary language of commerce and science around the world.

These factors made the usually difficult process of starting and staffing new educational institutions more efficient than elsewhere in Africa. One of the authors has had the opportunity to assist in the creation of completely new higher educational institutions in several African countries. The time to create a new institution in Rwanda, complete with legislation to recognize the new degree and then move the program to the capital city Kigali to make it more accessible to students and relevant to the country, was less than half that required in the other countries. This was primarily due to support at all levels of the Government and a lack of "old guard" academic opposition within the university system.

In the health area one of the first efforts in higher education was the creation of a School of Public Health assisted by Tulane University in order to provide graduate medical professionals trained in preventive as well as curative medicine. This institution became the first branch of the national University to locate in Kigali and to begin to offer technology-supported courses as envisioned in the national plan. The Kigali Institute of Health, a health oriented undergraduate institution based in Kigali provides much of the human resources for the growing health sector.

Rwanda is a good example of a country that is poised to benefit significantly from technology assisted distance education (which has begun at several universities) They are also trying to upgrade their university and graduate education sectors. The establishment of a science and technology University, the Kigali Institute of Technology, (KIST) as the first major supplement to the traditional National University of Rwanda in Butare was the first step in trying to provide the technical human resources to drive the vision of a knowledge-based economy in the heart of Africa.

Finally, under the early leadership of dynamic Ministry of Education, Romain Murenzi (a former U.S. university faculty member and Professor of Physics) and the current Minister of Science, Research and Technology, Rwanda established an aggressive policy of seeing assistance in higher education from institutions around the world. This assistance has come in the form of joint programs and faculty and student exchanges. While many African educational institutions are inwardly centered, the important efforts of educators and politicians in Rwanda to look outward with the ultimate goal of creating competitive institutions able to generate graduates world-class is notable.

With all of the positive changes in education, Rwanda still faces huge challenges in developing the needed cadre for higher education in the country. The process of developing senior researchers is slow and expensive (a PhD averages six to seven years from the end of undergraduate training). In the rush to achieve literacy and primary schooling, the needed quality control is not present and as a result the quality of the graduates is varied. While a policy commitment to technology assisted education is present at the highest levels the experience, equipment and implementing environment is still lacking. The decentralized performance based paradigm so effective in other areas has been less implemented in the educational arena where traditional institutions are still relatively strong. It is sorely needed.

Despite these challenges however education in Rwanda is a bright spot in Africa with at the potential for achieving major advances in the medium term. The vision and commitment of the senior policy leaders can make up for some of the lack of resources and low starting point from which Rwandan education has emerged.

Gender: Progress

I had to leave the baby with my husband. When I woke up, the troops had left. I needed to join them. I put on my uniform and ran outside. I jumped in an army truck and we started driving toward the front. On the way, we picked up other soldiers who had been left behind. We made it to the front. The fighting was fierce. Our lowest point came when we heard that both Fred (Rwigema) and Peter (Baingana) had died. Paul Kagame was in the United States. We had no leader. When he arrived things really started to turn around. We would not have survived without his leadership. One day when I was at the front, and the fighting was fierce, I looked at the person next to me. It was my husband. "Where is our baby," I asked? "I had to leave him with a village girl," he said.[8]

Women soldiers played a major—if largely unheralded and unexamined—role[9] in stopping the genocide[10] and have gone on to structure institutions and laws so that now to a degree unprecedented in any country in the world, women hold significant power in Rwanda.

In the September, 2008 Parliamentary elections, 56% of those elected were women. The world average for women in national Parliaments is 15.1%. Rwanda is the first country in the world where women outnumber men in Parliament .This is worth repeating. Rwanda now has more women in Parliament than any country in the world.[11] In one of the poorest countries in the world, one that was completely devastated by the 1994 genocide, women now control the Parliament and hold one-third of the Cabinet positions.

The recent elections built on progress that started in the early part of the decade. Near the end of the transitional period that lasted until 2003, a committee was established to draft the new Constitution. Three members of the constitutional Commission, a quarter of the total membership, were women. Major NGOs including the umbrella organization Collectifs Pro-Femmes/Twese Hamwe (Pro-Femmes) worked with the Minister of Gender and other NGOs to ensure that woman's voices and concerns were embedded in the new laws for the country. Article 10 of the Constitution reflects this commitment to gender equity:

> *We the People of Rwanda . . . Committed to ensuring equal rights between Rwandans and between women and men without prejudice to the principles of gender equality and complementality in national development.*

In the 2003 elections, 48.8% of Members of Parliament (MPs) were women. The 2008 elections built on that impressive early success to catapult Rwanda into first place in this important indicator of gender empowerment. Women also fill the Cabinet, the Ministries and the Office of the Presidency, including: Education, Foreign Affairs, Health, Gender, Labour, Environment, and Agriculture are women. The head of the Supreme Court and the Commissioner of Police are women. Numerous public institutions are headed by women including the powerful Rwanda Revenue Authority, REIPA, National Insurance, Tourism, National AIDS, Unity and Reconciliation and Human Rights Commissions, Gacaca, the Auditor-General, the Deputy Governor of the Bank, the Ombudsman, the French Commission and Rose Kabuye as the Chief of Protocol.

How did this happen in a traditional, patriarchal society? How have women come to hold such broad and deep positions of power and leadership and what does it mean for the future of the country?

The emphasis on women and gender equity is both philosophical and practical. Women were equally involved in the Rwandan Patriotic Front and those who grew up as exiles in Uganda were influenced by that country's quote system that reserves 20% of seats in Parliament to women.[12] Equally important, in the early post-genocide years in Rwanda, the majority of people in the country, close to 70% were female.

It is also very clear that the foundation for this commitment to gender equity is based in part on the powerful vision of President Paul Kagame. During discussions held to write the new constitution, he reminded the drafters of the role women played in stopping the genocide as well as the important role women could play in rebuilding the country.

In an interview in the summer of 2005, I asked him where this vision came from. He responded by asking me what I thought. I mentioned the role Rose Kabuye and many other women played in fighting to stop the genocide and asked him if this helped to shape his vision. It did he said.

He went on to say that representatives of academia and the international lending institutions had lectured him about the importance of gender in development and that really he had seen first hand that "women were equal in all ways to men."[13]

President Kagame's commitment to gender equity was reflected in 2007 when he won the African Gender Award for his support of gender equality. The award was granted by the Women African Solidarity (FAS) and the Committee of the African Women for Peace and Development (AWCPD) who said: "President Paul Kagame has made exceptional efforts to promote the rights of women in his country." In accepting that award, President Kagame said: "Today women constitute half of our population. . . . It is therefore an affront that decisions that affect their lives continue to be made without their participation."[14]

By far the greatest piece of legal text that changed life for women is the June 4, 2003 Constitution of Rwanda. The 2003 constitution mandates that a minimum of 30% seats is held by women for all decision-making levels in the government. The constitution established principles of equality for men and women in every aspect and mandatory representation of women at every level of leadership in the country.

Women legislators have already started to have a significant impact.[15] One of the most significant pieces of legislation drafted by women was the succession act that gave girls and women a right to inherit in Rwanda for the first time. Before legislation was passed during the transition period in 1999, only a male's offspring inherited from the father and if a man did not have sons, his brothers or male relatives would inherit. This legislation—which is enshrined in the constitution—also gives women a right to own property just like men. The law on immigration and citizenship also for the first time recognizes that children whose mothers are Rwandese are automatically Rwandese. Before this law was passed one was automatically Rwandan only if his/her father was Rwandese. If you had a Rwandan mother, you had to apply for citizen ship like any other foreigner. These laws are removing the barriers to full participation in all aspects of society, and may be the keys to why development in Rwanda is likely to be more sustainable than in many other poor countries.

Rwanda has taken another step that ensures that the gains in gender equity will be sustainable. The authors conducted a systematic review of textbooks used throughout the nation in the primary grades (1 through 6) to analyze how the genocide is presented. Much to our surprise we discovered multiple examples if exercises that show that young children in

Rwanda are being taught to examine traditional roles of men and women, and to discuss the importance of educating girls. The primary six text-book: *Macmillan Rwanda: Primary Social Studies* authored by four Rwandans: Emmanuel Bamusananire, Joseph Byiringiro, Augustine Munyakazi and Johnson Ntagaramga ends one chapter with this exercise:

Figure 4.1
Questions about Girls' Education

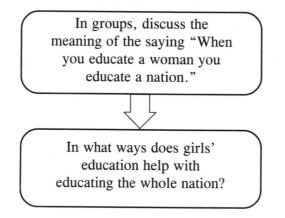

This same textbook has an in-depth discussion of traditional roles for men and women in Rwandan society. The textbook goes on to list them:

Figure 4.2
Gender in Our Province

The Traditional Place of Men and Women

Men

- Men were the most important people in the household.
- Men owned the land and the cattle.
- They were responsible for the family' income. Men carried out traditional trade exchanges.
- Only men could give a name to their child.
- Men were responsible for building the family house.
- Only men could plant trees for the family wood.
- All adult men or young boys could be chosen to spend time at the Royal Court or with the local chief. *(continued)*

Figure 4.2 (continued)
Gender in Our Province

Women

- Women were responsible for planting and harvesting food crops.
- Women did all the cooking and child care.
- Women carried water to the home and fetched firewood.
- Women were responsible for their family's health. They grew herbs and made medicines.
- Women were considered to be the peacemakers.

Men and women were treated differently in traditional Rwandan society.

Inheritance

Women were unable to inherit property or land. This meant that they were unable to provide for their children if their husband died However the brother-in-law or clan leader would make sure that widows and orphans were not discriminated against

Business

Traditional social law stopped women from running a business or working in any business without their husband's permission

Education

Traditional education for girls did not include formal schooling

Legal rights

The Civil Code and the Family Code stated hat the husband was the head of the household and that his will would be legally upheld in disagreements between husband and wife.

Figure 4.3
Traditional Roles for Men and Women

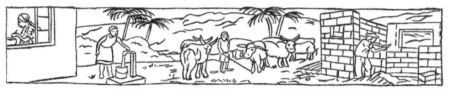

Activities

1. Read the text carefully
2. In groups, discuss the consequences for both women and men, of the traditional treatment of women. Are the points true for your province?
3. In your notebooks, draw two large circles and divide each into six segments. Write 'men' in the centre of one circle and 'women' in the centre of the other. Draw a symbol in each segment to show the different responsibilities of men and women in traditional society in your province.

Position of Men and Women in Our Province Today

- Women run businesses and are able to borrow from banks.
- Men are no longer assumed to be the head of a household. If a husband and wife divorce, the care of the children is decided by agreement.
- Women are now on committees at each level of government
- More men than women receive higher education

Activities

1. Read the points about the position of men and women today.
2. In your notebooks, make two columns with the headings Men/ Women. Write one or two words for each point. Add some more words to describe the position of men and women in your province.

Gender: Challenges

Rwanda has taken impressive steps to ensure gender empowerment. Gender equity at the primary school level was reached in 2000—fifteen years ahead of the MDG target. Women now constitute the majority of Parliamentarians. In local governments female representation increased from 28% in 2003 to over 40% in 2006. Women in decision-making positions in Rwanda have taken on significant challenges and the constitution and laws that have been passed to ensure equality will have a long term and important impact.

Despite this unprecedented progress, numerous challenges remain. Poverty has a female face in Rwanda. Because of the legacy of the genocide, a third of households are headed by single women and 62% of those households live below the poverty line. Illiteracy rates are higher for women than men (29 for women verses 22 for men) and women work primarily in the agricultural sector (86%) where poverty levels are the highest. A 2005 Demographic and Health Survey (DHS) documented that close to a third of women in Rwanda had suffered from physical violence. In 19% of the cases that violence had occurred in the previous year and in the majority of cases the abuse was caused by the husband or partner.[16]

The greatest challenge facing not just women but the entire country is rapid population growth. High levels of female fertility could overwhelm much of the progress not only in improving gender equity and empowerment but also other goals such as reducing poverty, increasing access to education, improving health, and reversing environmental destruction.[17]

Rwanda's leaders have long understood the challenges of rapid population growth and this issue figures prominently in the Vision 2020 planning document Vision 2020:

> [T]he Rwandan population has been characterised, during the last century, by a strong demographic growth without improvement in skills or economic and technological performances. This demographic trend is one of the main causes of the depletion of natural resources and the structural impoverishment of the population. Controlling demographic growth with regard to capacities for sustainable economic growth, the improvement of the health status and the building of the population's human capacities so as to make these become a true valuable resource

at the level of national and foreign markets, constitute a major challenge to be taken up by Rwanda.

The total fertility rate in Rwanda in 2007 was 6.1 children per woman increasing from 5.8 children per woman in 2000. The population growth rate is close to 3%.This high level means that Rwanda's population, currently estimated at around 8.9 million will double by 2030. Every time the population doubles, Rwanda must provide twice the infrastructure, twice the social services, and twice the production of basic needs, just to keep the standard of living from deteriorating. Unless policies are programs are developed quickly to reduce the fertility rate, this rapid growth could overcome all of the positive efforts to reduce poverty, increase educational levels and improve the overall quality of life in Rwanda.

There are some signs of progress. The desired fertility level is far below the current rate. According to a recent survey, women desire 4.3 children and men 4.0 children. This means that widespread access to modern contraception, could lead to a rapid reduction in the fertility rate and lower over time, the growth of the population. There is some data to indicate that this is already occurring: national survey data from 2008 show that the use of modern contraception (such as the pill, condoms, implants etc) increased from 17 percent in 2005 to 36 percent in 2008. That same survey shows that the infant mortality rate which measures the number of deaths per 1000 live births dropped from 86 in 2005 to 62 in 2008. This is a strong and important relationship between female fertility and infant and child mortality. When many babies are dying, women will continue to have large families until they see that more of their children live through childbirth. Child mortality, the mortality of children from age 1 to 5 also fell from 152 deaths/1000 in 2005 to 103/1000 in 2008.

Improving education for women and men in the area of reproductive health is also a priority. Rwanda remains a conservative society in issues of sex and reproductive health. "Our culture does not allow us to talk easily about sex or HIV/AIDS," said one educator. Vision 2020 in a surprisingly candid manner, also recognized the deeply ingrained cultural determinants of gender inequity:

The discrimination against women originates from the Rwandan culture and tradition, which consider the girl as inferior to the boy, physically, intellectually and socially. As such, the woman might be submitted to the man. The women benefit from the man's protection, but this tends to distance them from the ownership of properties and reduces their role in the management of the society.

The division of labour exempted them from tasks considered as heavy but, as a consequence, the civic merit and even the material wealth which were at the basis of Individuals' social status were kept out of their reach.

The advent of the Judaeo-Christian religion with colonisation has reinforced the woman in her position of inferiority and submission to the man. This is how Rwandan girls have far less benefited from schooling particularly schooling organised by religious groups: less access to formal education, drop-out rates clearly superior to those of boys, less subjects leading to profit making careers. . . . Rwanda endeavours to progressively rectify this situation but cultural inertia is hard to overcome and as such changes in terms of gender come very slowly. Nevertheless the woman must, as a human being, enjoy all her rights without discrimination, in conformity with the open will for social equity and serve her country according to her competencies as a human resource. The process towards equality and complementarity between the sexes risk being curbed by the passivity of the culture and traditions, by the low level of parents' education—especially with respect to mothers, by the parents' poverty, by other sorts of inequalities related to gender roles and by the attitude of religions and religious sects.[18]

Traditional gender roles continue to structure relations between men and women, and have an impact on educational access and attainment and improving health outcomes, especially in rural areas. Girls are still primarily responsible for household chores including such time consuming tasks as fetching water and firewood, and taking care of the sick, including those with HIV/AIDS. These roles and tasks often lead to absenteeism and withdrawal from school.

HIV/AIDS prevalence while low in the country at about 3% is higher among women than men (3.6 versus 2.3) and higher in urban than rural areas (7.3 versus 2.2). Only 54 percent of women and 50 percent of men have "comprehensive knowledge of HIV/AIDS, meaning they have correct information concerning methods of prevention and transmission. Among young women and men between the ages of 15-24, only half have "comprehensive knowledge" of HIV/AIDS."[19]

Despite unprecedented access to power and enormous strides in increasing access for girls to primary school, significant structural challenges remain, especially in increasing girl's access to secondary school and higher education, increasing the participation of girls studying math, science and technology, and improving completion rates at the primary and secondary level especially between rural and urban areas. The cost of education, combined with failure to pass the primary school exit exam are the two primary reasons cited by parents in a recent survey to determine why completion rates for girls are low. Both are affected by poverty and traditional gender roles. While poverty reduction is a priority for the government, widespread programs to sensitize the population to issues of gender equity (beyond the classroom) are essential. Moreover, improving girl's access to secondary school is an important goal in its own right but also one of the most significant predictors of declining fertility and improving childhood health over time.

Health

In 1994 most of Rwanda's infrastructure, including its health care facilities was destroyed. Those who survived the genocide were hungry and hurt. "There was no food to eat or any medicines. People grouped together to grow food and take care of each other," said Bonaventure about those first months after the genocide in Kigali.

Vision 2020 recognized how serious the health challenges were for the country:

> The level of the health status of the Rwandan population is insufficient. The prevalence of malaria (50% of consultations in health facilities) and HIV/AIDS (11.2% of the population as a whole) is high and constitutes, along with other health problems, a big socio-economic issue. The physically and mentally if not socially traumatised are many, due to the 1994 genocide. The health situation is a handicap to the country's economy and its future.[20]

From a very low base, Rwanda has made significant progress in recognizing the importance of health in development and in recent years improving important indicators of human health. They have introduced several innovations, including widening access to health care through community-based health insurance programs, and sophisticated monitoring and evaluation of health care programs, that when fully developed could be models for the rest of the continent.

According to the World Bank, at 96%, Rwanda now has one of the highest rates of immunization in Sub-Saharan Africa, and received the 2008 PACE (Pneumococcal Awareness Council of Experts) Global Leadership Award[21] for its groundbreaking efforts to introduce the pneumococcal vaccine in Rwanda. Infant mortality, the number of children dying per 1,000 live births, has decreased from a very high rate of 107/1000 in 1999 to 86/1000 in 2007. HIV prevalence has decreased from 13% immediately after the genocide to 3%, although remaining high for women in Kigali at 8.6% because of the legacy of rape occurring during the genocide. (As in other African countries part of this decrease is due to better measurement and assessment tools like those instituted by the Rwandan government) Access to health facilities has improved with 60% of Rwandans now living within 5 kilometers of a health facility and 85% within 10 kilometers.

Several innovative programs have contributed to these impressive improvements in health outcomes and improvements by making health care more affordable, accessible and results-oriented.

Like Gacaca that was modified to deal with perpetrators of the genocide, and Imihigo, revised to ensure that leaders are held accountable, Rwanda has reached back to a cultural tradition and expanded its scope in order to improve health outcomes. Mutuelle de Santé, a community-based health insurance plan that was started during the transitional period in 1999, draws on a centuries-old tradition of mutual aid programs that were prominent throughout many parts of Africa in the 18th and 19th centuries. These community-based health insurance schemes were prominent in Rwanda in the 1960s with Association Muvandimwe de Kibungo and Association Umubano Mubantu de Butare being the most prominent.[22]

Initially when Mutuelle de Santa was developed in 1999 it only operated in a small section of the country. Since 2004, mutual health insurance is countrywide and by 2008, 75% of Rwandans had health insurance. The goal in Rwanda is universal health coverage at an affordable rate.

How does Mutuelle de Santé work? Each member of the insurance program pays 1000 Rwandan francs for basic coverage (about $2); the government contributes a portion of the health budget to the insurance program and recently international donors and non-governmental organizations have also contributed. A district committee determines who is too poor to pay and has the authority to waive fees. It is estimated that 10% of the population in 2004 had their fees waived because of poverty. Those with HIV/AIDS who are in a PEPFAR program also do not pay for care through this program.

The programs are administered by their members who draw up a Constitution defining the structure, by-laws and management. They determine their premiums and packages and choose their service providers. Most of the programs use a family-based fee base with special rates for the very poor and vulnerable people (such as widows and orphans.) Packages can be purchased that include minimum coverage: pre- and postnatal consultations, nursing care, vaccinations, family planning, simple childbirth, essential and generic drugs laboratory analysis, minor surgical procedures, and transport to a hospital. More expanded coverage, called Complementary Coverage includes hospital care in district hospitals, consultation by a doctor, caesarian operations, minor and major surgical procedures, all diseases from 0-5 and laboratory analysis.[23]

To strengthen the financial viability of the program, in November 2008, three additional funds, the Social Security Fund of Rwanda, the medical insurance scheme, (RAMA) and the Military Medical Insurance were merged with Mutuelle de Santé. The International Social Security Association (ISSA) commended Rwanda for its innovative efforts to expand health care coverage saying, "It has significant increased health care in the country."[24]

Performance based contracting, discussed in chapter three, extends to the health sector. The improved pay and other incentives for health care workers in specific districts, at least according to preliminary research, shows positive improvements in health outcomes health provider's income is linked to improving those outcomes. For example, family planning coverage was 28 times greater in a district that had performance-based pay than compared to one that did not.

Connecting Technology to Health

Rwanda is a leader in using technology in innovative ways to improve health. TRACnet is a part of Rwanda's plan to use information technologies to reduce poverty and generate economic growth. TRAC, The Treatment and Research AIDS Center, has its origins in the National AIDS Control Program (NACP) that had responsibility for implementing nation-wide AIDS programs from 1987-2000. In 2000 this organization was restructured into two major units: one responsible for developing the policy framework and coordinating among sectors (National AIDS Control Commission), and a second unit TRAC was designed to improve care, decentralize health services and maintain research and surveillance.

TRACnet is charged with data collection, information sharing and monitoring and analysis of AIDS programs. It is innovative in its use of information technology by using allowing health professional to use mobile phones (and the Internet) both for submitting reports on HIV patients, tracking results and for accessing laboratory results.[25] Mobile phone use helps tremendously in areas without electricity or computers and Internet connections. In many parts of the developing world, even in poor countries like Rwanda, increasingly where there are people, there are mobile phones. Currently 85% of users input their data via mobile phones. 95% of all HIV/AIDS patients using anti-retrovirals in Rwanda are included in the tracking system.[26] This innovative program was developed in conjunction with the Government of Rwanda by the US Centers for Disease Control supported by Tulane University with software and technical assistance from a private company, Voxiva. TRACnet has received several global awards for its innovative use of technology including the United Nations Economic Commission for Africa (UNECA) award for "its efforts in improving the health of Rwandans through the use of information technology."

Health-Related Challenges

It is in using a broader definition of health, that includes measures of poverty such as nutritional status, that one gets a picture of the major challenges facing the government and people of Rwanda. Currently 56.9% of Rwandans live below the poverty line of $2 per day. 22.5% are malnourished and 36% do not have access to daily minimum calorie consumption.[27]

One of the major problems facing Rwanda, in all sectors is a dearth of highly qualified professionals. This is very evident in the health sector. Most districts have few nurses 1 for every 3,900 and fewer doctors, 2 per 100,000 inhabitants. There are few trained health professionals, including midwives in rural areas, thus contributing to an extremely high maternal mortality rate and high, though declining infant mortality rates. Malaria continues to be the main cause of childhood death in the country accounting for 35-40% of death in children under five years of age. The use of insecticide-treated bed nets, on of the proven interventions for reducing malaria, has increased nationwide from 4% in 2004 to 40% in 2006.

Water borne diseases remain prevalent. There has been some progress in this area access to clear water increasing to 14% in 2006. This has had a major impact on reducing child mortality, a 25% drop according to the World Bank.

While the government budget allocated to health has increased dramatically during the past decade, doubling from 2002 to 2004, the proportion allocated to the health sector, while it has increased from 6.1% in 2000 to 9.5% in 2007, is still low compared to the goal of 15% set by the government as well as the importance placed on good health in Vision 2020 and the Millennium indicators.

Rwanda shares problems faced by many African countries in having a large part of its national health budget focused on curative rather than preventive care and much of its programmatic financing supported by external donors. These funds often bring with them agendas and ideas from less than informed or qualified individuals who administer vertical or internationally funded (e.g. World Bank, World Health Organization) health funds. Generally when faced with the dilemma of accepting large blocs of funding with all sorts of strings attached or losing the money, developing countries will accept without condition the mandate of the outside agencies.

Rwanda has demonstrated time and time again that it is capable of not only judging the appropriateness of international funding but also insisting that development partners and international employees working in Rwanda are appropriate and knowledgeable about programs. Rwanda's leaders have succeeded in exerting high-level pressure and actually having individuals ejected because they were not knowledgeable and sensitive to national priorities. A leader in this process has been Dr. Agnes Binagwaho who served for many years as the Director of the National AIDS Committee, and was recently promoted to be the Minister of Health in charge of HIV/AIDS. The HIV/AIDS arena is particularly contentious regarding international funding because of the huge economic presence of international programs driven by PEPFAR, the World Bank and Global Fund. Dr. Binagwaho has implemented a national research review committee, which could become a model for Africa. Made up of Rwandan health experts it reviews research and action protocols, to avoid duplication and increase quality.[28] With the support of the Ministry of

Health, Dr. Binagwaho also expanded the extremely well funded HIV/AIDs area into a reformed TRAC plus unit, which includes active programs in Tuberculosis and Malaria as well as outbreak investigation, and related areas. By undertaking this structural and organizational change Rwanda has opened the path for using capacity building and infrastructure-oriented outside funding to cover some of the major diseases in the country and therefore help to avoid a skewed national health budget with respect to programmatic focus.

At the most senior levels, Rwanda has very highly skilled and competent public health professionals. This is not always the case, however at the regional and local levels. TRACNET was unable to recruit sufficiently well trained individuals to implement software and drug distribution programs, and as a result the implementation process has been delayed.

With all of these challenges, in this sector as in all areas, Rwanda has an appropriate plan and is trying to make the best use of available resources and create additional resources. The government does need to follow even more closely the link between health and development with particular attention to the nutrition issue, as well as the important aspects of mental and social well being need to be systematically addressed. Finally, the creation of an objectives based monitoring and evaluation system based on health outcomes is critical.

Notes

1. FAWE Rwanda Celebrates its 10th Anniversary, FAWE Rwanda Newsletter, December 2006. FAWE Rwanda "Speak Out Process," 2005, FAWE Rwanda Newsletter (January-April, 2007).

2. Government of Rwanda, Education Strategy Paper 2004, pp. 1-2.

3. International Monetary Fund. Rwanda: Joint Staff Assessment of the Poverty Reduction Strategy Paper (PRSP) Progress Report, August 2004, p. 4.

4. Republic of Rwanda, Self Evaluation: Education Sector, 2006. P 4.

5. Huggins, Allison and Shirley Randell. "Gender Equality in Education in Rwanda: What is Happening to our Girls?" Paper presented at the South African Association of Women Graduates Conference on "Dropouts from School and Tertiary Studies," Capetown, South Africa May, 2007.

6. Republic of Rwanda, Economic Development and Poverty Reduction Strategy 2008-2012, p. 3.

7. World Bank *Education in Rwanda: Rebalancing Resources to Accelerate Post-Conflict Development and Poverty Reduction.* Washington, D.C.: The World Bank, 2004Provides a good summary of the challenges faced in 1994 in the education sector and progress through 2003.

8. Interviews with (Retired) Lt. Colonel, Chief of Protocol, Office of the President, Rose Kabuye, 2005-08.

9. Izabiliza, Jeanne "The Role of Women in Reconstruction: Experience of Rwanda." Unpublished paper.

10. Rose Kabuye was one of the most senior women in the army, and is now the Chief of Protocol for President Kagame. Her story will be told in a forthcoming book, edited by Dr. Ensign.

11. See Devlin, Claire and Robert Elgie." The Effect of Increased Women's Representation in Parliament: The Case of Rwanda." *Parliamentary Affairs* Vol. 61 Issue 2 (April, 2008): 237-254, and Mutume, Gumisai. "Women Break Into African Politics." *Africa Recovery* Vol. 18, No. 1 (April 2004): 1-6.

12. Uganda also established a National Gender Policy in 1997, one of the first on the continent and in the 1995 Constitution established seats in Parliament for women by district. For an excellent case study see: Sylvia Tamale, *When Hens Begin to Crow: Gender and Parliamentary Politics in Uganda.* Boulder: Westview Press, 1999.

13. Interview with President Paul Kagame, July 2005.

14. Munyaneza, James. "Kagame Wins 2007 Africa Gender Award." AllAfrica.com January 28, 2007.

15. Devlin, Claire and Robert Elgie." The Effect of Increased Women's Representation in Parliament: The Case of Rwanda." *Parliamentary Affairs* Vol. 61 Issue 2 (April, 2008): 237-254; Elizabeth Pawley, *Rwanda: The Impact of Women Legislators on Policy Outcomes Affecting Children and Families.* Background Paper: The State of the World's Children, 2007 New York, UNICEF; Jennifer Brea. "The New Rwanda." *The Guardian,* 16 July 2007.

16. *Demographic and Health Survey: Rwanda.* Calverton, Maryland: ORC Macro, 2006.

17. Nyangara, Florence, Camilee Hart, Ilene Speizer and Scott Moreland. *Unmet Need for Family Planning in Rwanda and Madagascar: An Analysis Report for the Repositioning of Family Planning Initiatives.* Chapel Hill, Carolina Population Center, University of North Carolina, April, 2007.

18. Republic of Rwanda, Ministry of Finance and Economic Planning. Rwanda Vision 2020, 2000, p. 198.

19. *Demographic and Health Survey: Rwanda.* Calverton, Maryland: ORC Macro, 2006, Executive Summary.

20. Republic of Rwanda, Ministry of Finance and Economic Planning. Rwanda Vision 2020, 2000, p. 28.

21. "Rwanda Receives 2008 PACE Global Leadership Award." All africa.com 24 October 2008.

22. See Mladovsky, Philipa and Elias Mossialos. "A Conceptual Framework for Community-Based Health Insurance in Low-Income Countries: Social Capital and Economic Development." *World Development* Vol. 36, No. 4 (2008): 590-607; and USAID. "Twubakane Decentralization and Health Program Rwanda Report #12" October-December 2007; Robert Soeters, Christian Habineza and Peter Bob Peerenboom. "Performance-Based Financing and Changing the District Health System: Experience from Rwanda." *Bulletin of the World Health Organization* Vol. 84 No. 11 (November, 2006): 884-89; and Robert Soeters, and L. Musabgo Comparison of Two Output Schemes in Butare and Cyangugu Provinces with two Control Provinces in Rwanda, 2005 World Bank: *Global Partnership on Output-Based Aid* (GPOBA).

23. Republic of Rwanda, Ministry of Health. Mutual Health Insurance Policy in Rwanda December, 2004, P. 8.

24. "Rwanda: Pension Bodies Laud Country's Health Insurance." allAfrica.com 19, November 2008.

25. William Bertrand, "Progress and Challenges in Health Care and Information Technology in Rwanda." Presented at the Post-Genocide Rwanda Conference, California State University, Sacramento, CA. November 2-3, 2007. and PEPFAR (President's Emergency Plan for AIDS Relief) : Rwanda TRACnet enhances monitoring of ART Scale Up" www.pepfar.gov February, 2006.

26. Republic of Rwanda, Ministry of Health, The Center for the Treatment and Research on HIV/AIDS and Malaria, Tuberculosis and other epidemics. www.moh.gov.rw/docs/trac+presentation.pdf.

27. International Monetary Fund. *Final Evaluation Report of Rwanda's Poverty Reduction Strategy*, July, 2006 and Republic of Rwanda, Economic Development and Poverty Reduction Strategy 2008-2012.

28. She was also responsible for the rejection of a CDC Chief of Party who was judged not experienced enough for work in Rwanda. He had no African experience, no appropriate language skills and little appropriate management experience.

Chapter Five

Is Economic Growth Pro-Poor?

"More than a decade after the genocide, the tiny African nation has reemerged as a mecca for American entrepreneurs seeking redemption and profits alike. Rwanda is home to one of the most hopeful, if little noticed transformations in the bottom-line world of business. An African killing field, roughly the size of Vermont, turning into a mecca for venture capitalists."[1]

Heritage Foundation/Wall Street Journal Index of Economic Freedom recognizes Rwanda as the most improved country in Africa over the past ten years and seventh most improved in the world, in terms of economic freedom.[2]

ForgeAhead, an independent ICT research and consulting firm announces that President Kagame is the winner of African Lifetime Achievers Award in ICT

Kigali Institute of Science and Technology (KIST) wins the infoDev award from the World Bank for promoting Business Incubation in Rwanda.

Fast Company chooses Kigali as one of their 12 Fast Cities around the world that are thriving. With Rwanda's economy zipping along—growth has climbed past 6%—development dollars have flooded Kigali. A stock exchange opened in January, and President Paul Kagame has plans to build the capital into an African science-and-tech hub, pledging to spend 5% of GDP on research by 2012 and turning military facilities into educational ones.

Rwanda: One of the Top 29 Reformers Globally[3]

A s the headlines attest, the positive stories about Rwanda's economic, political and social recovery are beginning to emerge. Vision 2020 sets an ambitious goal for Rwanda to become a middle income-developing country by 2020. Parts of the vision are beginning to be realized. Beginning from the lowest possible base, the economy has experienced two stages of strong economic growth. During the transition period from 1996 to 2000, the economy grew on average at 10% per year. An evaluation of the UK's development programs in Rwanda from 2000-2006 concluded:

> There is general consensus that the results obtained during the first decade after genocide, have been remarkable. All the MDG indicators were dramatically reversed during the genocide and fell below 1990 levels. This reversal was compounded by the already existing structural constraints of a landlocked country, a low natural resource base, high transport costs, limited land availability and a high population growth rate. Despite these impediments, Rwanda has achieved impressive progress and has put in place crucial policies for pro-poor growth. After high growth in the initial rebound between 1995 and 2001, Rwanda managed to achieve real GDP growth of 6% to 10% in the three years up to 2003. There has been some diversification of exports and privatisation is being pursued energetically. The Government and the President of the Republic have a legitimate power base with widespread popular support.[4]

As the economy began to stabilize in the second phase, from 2001-06, growth remained strong averaging 6.5% per.[5] Export growth has also improved with growth rates of 12% per year since 2001. In 2006, Rwanda exported $152 million of exports double that of 2002. The primary exports are traditional ones—coffee, tea and pyrethrum (a natural insecticide), which contribute over 60% of exports. Horticulture has recently taken off with exports growing to the European Union.[6]

Value-added, fully washed coffee, which brings in increased revenues, saw a doubling from 5% of total coffee production in 2005 to 10% in 2006. Rwanda's coffee sector, which employs about 400,000 people, is slowly modernizing with large coffee producers such as Starbucks considering Rwandan coffee among the highest quality in the world.[7]

Coffee has always played an extremely important part in Rwanda's economy, but most of the infrastructure was devastated in the genocide.

The successful recovery of the coffee industry is a story that involved the US government represented by the US Agency for International Development (USAID) the Rwandan government and the private sector in the US, first with the Community Coffee Company of Baton Rouge, Louisiana and more recently, Starbucks. These have been very successful partnerships: coffee is now Rwanda's major export crop, representing 75% of export income. Rwandan coffee is now considered by many experts to be among the highest quality in the world. In 2007 the mega-coffee retailer Starbucks sold out the "Rwandan Blue Bourbon" brand in 5,000 of its shops.

The USAID component began with a project that trained farmers to grow high quality coffee beans and to renovate the coffee-washing stations. The project also helped the farmers to organize into cooperatives, pointed them to financing opportunities and introduced them to U.S. coffee retailers like Starbucks. According to the director of the USAID portion of the project, "this market-oriented partnership has improved the livelihoods of 40,000 Rwandan farmers by enabling them to sell a high-value crop, and is a perfect example of a successful partnership."

Do the small farmers benefit from this partnership? Do they get a fair portion of their product? How much of the $3.00 latte goes to the farmers? One of the authors spent a day with the Director of the Coffee Board in Rwanda, Ephram Niyonsaba, visited a washing station and learned about how Starbucks operates in Rwanda. Ephram told me that if those who purchase the coffee beans from the farmers receive a higher than expected price, they must pass on a percentage of the additional profit to the farmers. This is a very unusual practice.

For Starbucks, coffee and farmer equity or (C.A.F.E.) Practices are the heart of their framework: Basically, coffee producers are given a set of environmental and social criteria (quality and transparency are prerequisites). They are measured on their implementation of the criteria. Starbucks also has social development programs in the country focused on schools and health clinics as well as providing access to affordable credit to the farmers. The farmers are the focus here in Rwanda and lifting them out of poverty through income producing projects is the goal. This is a success story for all involved—the Rwandan government, the US government and the private sector.

Local Rwandans have also started growing and marketing their own coffee. Bourbon Coffee opened a now very popular coffee shop in downtown Kigali in 2007 (complete with wireless) and by 2008 was exporting its coffee overseas. In late 2008 it opened its first coffee shop in the US in a store vacated by Starbucks in Washington D.C.

While exports of tea and coffee have increased, these products are dependent upon fluctuating international prices, and do not offer a stable source of foreign exchange. According to the Ministry of Finance, "Although both the volume and value of Rwandan coffee exports rose during 2006, Rwanda was not able to take full advantage of these increased prices on international markets. In the first half of 2006 world prices for coffee were falling June offering the lowest price. This low coincided with the heights of Rwanda's coffee exports. Therefore the majority of the crop was not sold at a time conducive to gaining the higher prices seen at the end of 2006.)[8] Moreover, while modernizing these sectors is important, the majority of the population is not involved in growing tea and coffee. A major challenge for Rwanda is to reach subsistence farmers, increase their incomes and productivity.

Lonely Planet Travel Guide names Rwanda among its top 10 countries to visit in 2009.

As tourists from around the world begin to flock to Rwanda to see some of the world's few remaining great gorillas, tourism has begun to contribute a larger share to GDP. In 2002, few visited the country and receipts from tourism were only $5 million. By 2006 that figure had increased to $33 million and is likely to continue to increase rapidly with the rehabilitation of the national parks and the development of ecolodges in several party of the country. Dubai World, a private company based in the Emirate of Dubai, has invested over $230 million in a new lodge and golf resort. However, the impact of the new global recession may have very negative consequences for tourism.

The Office of Tourism and National Parks (ORTPN) sector was restructured in 2003 and has made significant progress not only increasing revenue, generating employment, (over 250,000 people work directly in the tourist sector, according to ORPTN), also developing innovative projects in the local communities. ORTPN was a fully funded government organization until 2005 when it became self-sufficient and revenue generating both for the central government as well as local communities. In fact, 5% of the revenue from the tourism sector goes back to community projects. The revenue has funded water collection tanks, employed ex-poachers who are now guides in the parks and has even funded a community lodge near the famous gorilla naming area. This sector has the potential to expand and generate significant revenue in Rwanda. "From a negligible base of less than US $5 million in 2002, Rwanda's Tourism Sector is expected to reach US $100 million in revenues by 2012, representing a compounded annual growth rate of over 40%. An estimated cumulative 280,000 jobs will be created in the process."[9]

Growth depends upon stable sources of energy and until recently Rwanda has had to depend on costly imports. In 2008 however, the first methane gas from Lake Kivu—where an estimated 65 million m3 of usable methane resides—began to be extracted. Not only could this gas provide Rwanda with needed natural has for industry, it could when modified, provide enough electricity for the entire country as well as an important and needed source of foreign exchange when exported to surrounding countries.[10]

Rwanda has worked hard to establish the laws and policies necessary for sustained growth and foreign investment. The World Bank and corporate rating systems such as Fitch Ratings have commended Rwanda's commitment to economic reform, good governance and macroeconomic stability. The World Bank's Country Policy and Institutional Assessment (CIP) rating increased from 3.5 in 2005 to 4.0 in 2006, out of a total of 6. All of Rwanda's efforts to establish an open economy are paying off. Investments are flowing in telecommunications; construction foreign investors have recently discovered Rwanda. While total foreign investment remains small, it is increasing rapidly. Reducing the cost of doing business in Rwanda is a high priority. Currently, Rwanda has the highest costs (transport, energy and communication) in the region, at nearly three times higher in Rwanda than in Tanzania or Kenya. In 2006 the authors tried to facilitate the export of pencil machinery and "pencil seconds" to Rwanda to begin a small sector devoted to manufacturing school supplies. Even though the "pencil seconds" were to be donated by a businessman in California who produced them in Thailand, the cost to ship the pencils from Mombasa to Kigali were higher than the cost from Thailand to Mombasa, and made the project too costly. Reducing transport costs is a high priority.

On January 31, 2008 a stock exchange was opened in Kigali. Initially it is only open to Rwandan companies but it is envisioned that over time foreign companies will be listed and able to invest in Rwandan companies. A dozen American investors who traveled with one of the authors to the region in November 2008 are seriously examining the possibility of investing in Rwandan companies.

In July 2007 Rwanda was admitted as a full member of the East African community, opening up a market of close to 1000 million people. A year later, in July 2008, President Kagame was elected Chairman of the EAC. Membership in the EAC is likely to provide numerous benefits including harmonizing trade and tax systems, and labor can now flow without restrictions among the member's countries potentially leading to improving skill base in Rwanda. A common tariff has been established with Tanzania, Kenya and Uganda that will increase government revenue.

Role of Information and Communications Technology (ICT)

To pull the country out of poverty and to become the information-technology hub for East and Central Africa, Rwanda envisions using ICTs in all sectors—education, health care, governance, tourism, agriculture and business. The Rwandan Information Technology Authority or RITA was established in 2002 by an act of Parliament as a high-powered think-tank with the mission of structuring the process and implementing the plans that will lead to an information society. It is responsible for advising the Government on all technologies and processes. Two plans have been developed by RITA; National Information and Communications NICI One and II. An ICT Park, the Kigali ICT Park is connected RITA and is becoming a center of innovation, production and showcase of ICT. The ICT Park offers companies office space and other services at a minimal cost. It contains a business incubator where ideas are nurtured and grown into ICT businesses with a range of support services including: technical, administrative, legal and access to venture capital.

The plans are thoughtful blueprints for using ICT to leapfrog into the digital world, but the country has a long way to go to complete nationwide implementation. Low cost, high-speed Internet access is not yet available, resulting in a costly dependence on satellite connectivity. An undersea cable that is expected to connect all of East Africa to broadband connectivity will give Rwanda and the region access to low-cost international connectivity is expected to be operational in late 2009. SEACOM the undersea high-bandwidth cable provider, announced in the summer of 2009 that the land infrastructure needed to connect with the fibre data cable had been completed and that testing of the network has begun. High speed and inexpensive bandwidth will open up the world of knowledge and business to Eastern and Southern Africa.

Plans are also underway to use biotechnology to improve crop yields, and science-based solutions to establish irrigation projects, clear water and energy. Laptops are being distributed to students in rural and urban primary schools, and once the undersea cable is completed in 2009, Rwanda will install a fiber optic backbone that will—over time—allow countrywide connectivity. When completed, the goal is to connect all of the government agencies in Kigali and the districts, as well as universities and schools, hospitals, private companies, and over time, individual households.

Already 12 pilot telecenters are working in the rural areas that include phones, faxes, Internet connectivity, photocopiers and scanners. E-governance projects are underway and the health sector has received several awards for its innovative technology-based tracking system.

One of the most interesting uses of technology—not unique to Rwanda—but implemented at the highest level is the aggressive use of cell phones and electronic messages to manage the country. Every key person in the Government has the number of all high level individuals important to his or her functioning in their cell and communicates regularly to verify and or otherwise manage problems. These ambitious efforts are being coordinated through RITA and the Minister of Science, Technology and Research. "Rwanda will integrate science and technology into all sectors of the economy," says Minister Murenzi.[11] He recognizes the tremendous challenges that face Rwanda, acknowledging the need for more trained scientists, teachers and university professors.

President Kagame has kept this vision at the forefront of the country's development policy:

> The application of science and technology is fundamental, and indeed indispensable to economic transformation of our country. Productive capacities in modern economies are not based merely on capital, land and labour. They are also dependent on scientific knowledge and sustained technological advances.

By articulating an information technology based development strategy and creating government institutions to implement that policy Rwanda has become a technology leader in Sub-Saharan Africa and a model for all developing countries. In fact, it is one of the few countries in the region and indeed the world to have a coherent national policy that links ICT to national development.

Kigali Institute of Science and Technology

KIST was established in November 1997, in a former military barracks, as a project of the United National Development Program (UNDP) and the government of Rwanda. KIST faculty and students have developed many usable and award winning products and projects to reduce poverty. In 2005, KIST won the Ashen Award for sustainable energy for its development of biogas digesters, which have been introduced into schools prisons, as well as the 2001 award for developing an oven that uses 25% of the fuel required by traditional ovens. Its entrepreneurship incubator works with the best graduates for one year providing them the intellectual and financial support needed to nurture small businesses.

KIST is a great example of a university developing applied programs to solve societal problems and is one that could be emulated around the developing (and developed) world.

Challenges

While the economy is growing has this growth benefited the poor? The majority of the poor (90%) live in rural areas and are engaged in subsistence farming. Growth in this sector, by definition is pro-poor. While Rwanda has made significant progress in growing its economy, because of rapid population growth and low productivity in agriculture, poverty has only been slightly reduced. While the economy has begun a structural transformation from agriculture to services, serious challenges remain. Rapid population growth is putting increasing pressures on already fragile land. Rwanda has the highest population growth rate in Sub-Saharan Africa combined with the highest population density in the world.

According to the World Bank poverty indicators based on caloric consumption have fallen from 2000 to 2006 but very modestly. Rapid population growth and low productivity in agriculture means that while at the national level poverty has decreased from 60.4% to 56.9% from 2000 to 2006, because of population growth the numbers of poor people increased from 4.8 million to 5.3 million in 2006. Poverty is highest among those working in the agricultural sector with 91.2% living below the poverty line. Food insecurity remains a very serious problem with 52% of households in the country suffering from hunger and insecurity.

While Rwanda's economic growth rates were above the average growth rates for most of Sub-Saharan Africa they are below the Vision 2020 and PRSP targets and they also hide tremendous variation from year to year. Rwanda's economy is still primarily dependent upon agriculture and in Rwanda, like in many Sub-Saharan countries, agriculture is dependent upon rainfall. When the rains fail, agriculture suffers, and this is exactly what happened in 2006: "The rains were significantly below their seasonal averages. Most crops failed to stay at their 2005 levels and the overall volume of crops reduced by 2.1 percent." The Ministry of Agriculture, (MINAGRI) calculates that 33,000 tones (cereal equivalent) of food aid were needed in 2006. This dependency on rainfall is one of the primary causes of hunger and food security. Establishing a countrywide irrigation system is essential if hunger and poverty are to be reduced.

There has been no Green Revolution in Africa. The high yielding seeds and new farming techniques that were introduced first in Asia in the 1960s then in every region of the world except Africa resulted in very significant improvements in food security. New seeds and farming techniques as well as irrigation are essential to reduce poverty on a wide scale. Extending credit as well as research results to farmers will also contribute to improved production and poverty reduction.

The level of technology use in agriculture is low and infrastructure is poor. The Ministry of Finance in its 2006 Annual Economic Report indicates that only 3% of households use improved seeds and that fertilizer use is very low.[12] Rwanda would benefit from a system similar to one adopted by the U.S., which created the structure for the United States to become the world's leader in agricultural production. The Land Grant College System established in the mid-1800s as an Act of Congress led to a system of nation wide education and research universities dedicated to getting up to date information to the people who raised the food. In 1914 the Smith–Lever act mandated that each State university should have an extension agent who was dedicated to taking the tools of agricultural research and distributing the results among the population. Much of the original entrepreneurial and innovation research in the US sprang from these roots, with the research and new innovations from the Land Grant universities being transmitted to communities through agricultural extension agents. Using new information technologies, a county agent operating in this environment could assist with rapid transformation of the sector resulting in improved agricultural productivity and reduced malnutrition.

Rural roads and infrastructure, two of the major constraints in this area, are being improved, and there has been some increase in the use of fertilizer (organic and chemical fertilizer use has doubled from 2000-2006). Major land reform legislation was passed in 2005. The Land Law ensures that land is registered, and encourages land consolidation. Securing property rights should lead to increased access to credit for farmers and this increased investment should stimulate production and reduce poverty. The fragmentation of land into small plots has been one of the constraints in poverty reduction and in improving agricultural productivity. Government statistics show that "more than 60% of households cultivate less than 0.7 ha of land, and more than a quarter cultivate less than 0.2 ha."[13] In fact households are encouraged to consolidate their plots to ensure that holdings are not less than 1 hectare. Local (ubudehe) surveys conduced nationwide in 2006[14] identify lack of land as one the major causes of poverty along with soil erosion.

An additional cause for concern is the increasing income inequality in the country. The Gini coefficient (a measure of income inequality) deteriorated from 2000 to 2006. Economic growth is primarily helping those living in urban areas that have better access to employment, health care and education. Moreover, the country is heavily dependent upon foreign assistance, which averages about 20% of GDP. That is high compared to other countries in the region.

Rwanda's vision is to transform the country from one based on agriculture to an information and knowledge-based economy. It is a visionary goal, and perhaps one of the only ways poor countries can join the league of middle-income countries in our increasingly information-based globalized world. Yet Rwanda remains one of the poorest countries in the world with the majority of its population living in absolute poverty. Its economy is still primary based on agriculture. The country's leaders recognize that poverty has not been reduced as much as planned and have formulated another innovative program at the local level designed to reduce rural poverty.

Table 5.1
Causes of Poverty

Major Causes of Poverty	Share of Respondents (%)
Lack of land (Kutagira isambu)	49.5
Poor soils (Ubutaka butera)	10.9
Drought/weather (Izuba ryinshi)	8.7
Lack of livestock (Kutagira itungo)	6.5
Ignorance (Ubujiji)	4.3
Inadequate infrastructure (Ibikorwa remezo bidahagije)	3.0
Inadequate technology (Ikoranabuhanga ridahagije)	1.7
Sickness (Uburwayi)	1.7
Polygamy (Ubuharike)	1.2
Lack of access to water (Kubura amazi)	1.1
Population pressure (Ubwiyongere bw'abaturage)	0.7
Others(Izindi)	10.6
TOTAL	**100**

Turning to Local Solutions

Imihigo, a community-based statement of needs developed through Ubudehe and communicated to an elected official, who commits to meeting these needs, is likely to improve the lives of the poor over time—as resources are matched with needs of the poor. Yet another program has emerged that has the potential to offer faster reductions in poverty, especially absolute poverty. Called Vision 2020 Umurenge (VUP): An Integrated Local Development Program to Accelerate Poverty Eradication, Rural Growth and Social Protection, it is an explicit acknowledgement that poverty reduction has not occurred as rapidly as planned, that relying on economic growth alone is far from sufficient.

Evidence from a number of surveys conducted in Rwanda over the past few years give strong indication on the scale and depth of poverty. The Household Living Conditions Survey (EICV) indicates that the poverty rate was still 57% in 2005/06 with a poverty line at RwF 250 per adult and per day (or RwF 90,000 per adult and per year). This represents less than ½ dollar a day at current exchange rate.

Worse still, the extreme poverty rate stood at 37% in 2005/06; this indicates that more than 1 Rwandan in 3 cannot afford the minimum food basket of 2,500 kcal per adult per day, priced at RwF 175 per adult per day (or RwF 63,000 per adult and per year). The average income of the poor is RwF 150 per adult per day and most poor, who live in subsistence, do not even have such money in cash.[14] As anecdotal evidence, surveyors found that many poor people could not afford the RwF 10 user fee for water, one of the most basic necessities in life, and had no other choice but walking several kilometers to fetch soiled water and eventually contaminate their family. Income poverty is not the only indicator available. The Comprehensive Food Security and Vulnerability Analysis (CFSVA) indicate that 52% of households in Rwanda are either food insure or vulnerable. . . .

Almost half (43%) of the Rwandan population in under the age of 15 and 45% of children under the age of 5 suffer from chronic malnutrition, 19% suffer from its most severe form. Worse still, 55% of children aged 12-23 month are stunted, thereby hampering their future body growth.[15]

Vision 2020 Umurenge (VUP) has three primary goals:

1. To generate income and employment at the local level through public works. These projects are identified using the existing community-based planning approaches, such as Ubudehe and Community Development Forums. Projects that are underway include: watershed management, terracing, water harvesting, irrigation, feeder/access roads construction, building of classrooms, health facilities, training centers, business workshops, and village settlements.

2. To provide credit to farmers for necessary inputs like fertilizer and seeds and to create small businesses. Most households in the subsistence or informal sectors (i.e. about 2/3 of the Rwandan economy) seldom have access to capital or for-

mal credit; only 4.1% of domestic credit to the economy
went to agriculture, animal husbandries and fisheries in
2002-06.
3. To provide direct support for landless households. This portion would support the most vulnerable in the population—
widows, orphans and includes direct supports to improve
access to social services or to provide for landless households with no members qualifying for public works or credit
packages.

VUP began with two pilots in the fall of 2008 and through 2009 is being
extended to the 30 poorest communities in the country. A more radical
solution to rural poverty, grouping people together in planned communities that would improve access to education, health care, micro-credit is
being considered.

Rwanda has a long way to go to reach its Vision 2020 economic
goals. Growth has increased, but because of rapid population growth,
poverty remains very high and the land is under increasing stress. But
new programs have been designed, new targets for poverty reduction
established, and hope is high in the country. Hope is hard to quantify but
this is part of what makes Rwanda unique: the ability to move forward
with a positive attitude to, as Minister Musoni says, "create conditions
which can lead to a significant empowerment of those who at present
have little control over the forces that condition their lives."[16]

The bank is doing well. We have backers from India. The economy is
growing. I never thought I would look out at the hills of Kigali and see
so many lights. Rwanda is reborn.

—Bonaventure Niyibizi, November 2008

Notes

1. CNNMoney.com 2007.
2. *Wall Street Journal*, Heritage Foundation Index, 2006.
3. World Bank, *Doing Business 2008*.

4. Department for International Development, UK: Evaluation of DFID Country Program: Country Study Rwanda 2000-2006. Evaluation Report EV 60, January, 2006, p. 6.

5. Republic of Rwanda, Ministry of Finance and Economic Planning (2007) EDPRS Poverty Analysis of Ubudehe, Republic of Rwanda, Kigali, pp. 15-17.

6. See Government of Rwanda REIPA Annual Report, 2007.

7. *New York Times*, "Coffee and Hope Grow in Rwanda." April 6, 2006; USAID, "USAID and Rwandan Ambassador Celebrate Rwanda Coffee." Press Release, April 11, 2006.

8. Republic of Rwanda, Ministry of Finance and Economic Planning (2007) EDPRS. P. 10.

9. International Monetary Fund. *Final Evaluation Report of Rwanda's Poverty Reduction Strategy, 2006*, p. 37.

10. See "Rwanda: Road to Prosperity, Special Supplement." *The Independent*, August 1-7, 2008.

11. Interview with Minister Murenzi, July 2007. Also see "Africa in the Global Knowledge Economy,' In *Going for Growth: Science, Technology and Innovation in Africa*, edited by Calestous Juma, 2005.

12. See Government of Rwanda Vision 2020 Umurenge: An Integrated Local Development Program to Accelerate Poverty Eradication, Rural Growth and Social Protection." EDPRS Flagship Program Document, August, 2007; Republic of Rwanda, Economic Development and Poverty Reduction Strategy 2008-2012; Republic of Rwanda, Ministry of Finance and Economic Planning: Annual Economic Reports, 2005-07; Republic of Rwanda, Ministry of Finance and Economic Planning. National Microfinance Policy, September, 2006; and Republic of Rwanda, Ministry of Finance and Economic Planning (2007) EDPRS Poverty Analysis of Ubudehe, Republic of Rwanda, Kigali.

13. Republic of Rwanda, Economic Development and Poverty Reduction Strategy 2008-2012, p. 9.

14. Republic of Rwanda, Economic Development and Poverty Reduction Strategy 2008-2012, p. 14.

15. Government of Rwanda Vision 2020 Umurenge: An Integrated Local Development Program to Accelerate Poverty Eradication, Rural Growth and Social Protection." EDPRS Flagship Program Document, August, 2007, p. 8.

16. Interview with Minister Protais Musoni, July 2007.

Summary and Conclusion

How far has Rwanda come since 1994? Is there enough evidence to say that real progress is occurring in democracy and governance, in improving basic needs especially in education, health and gender equity, and in pro-poor economic growth?

Contrary to public perception and conventional wisdom, Rwanda has made tremendous progress since 1994 in all of these areas. It has more women in Parliament than any country in the world, and is committed to gender equity in all areas of society. Nine years of schooling are free, and enrollment is high and growing. The health care system is using information technology in creative ways to reach people and track their health status. People are participating and are elected freely at all levels of government and politics. The poor are determining their own needs and with the support of the government, and international donors, especially the European Union, have developed models that could be replicated in any poor country in the world. Ubudehe and Imihigo are country-wide, comprehensive and successful. Leaders are being held accountable for decisions through Imihigos. The poor are participating and running for office. The economy, though small, is growing and the discovery of natural gas will help fuel not only Rwanda's economy but those of neighboring countries as well. Much of the country will be wired for the Internet by the end of 2009, opening up the world's knowledge to the entire population. The country is secure and stable. Participants in the genocide are being held accountable.

Of course many challenges remain. The high rate of population growth could overwhelm efforts to educate all children through primary school as well as reduce the impact of poverty reduction programs. The global economic downturn that began in the fall of 2008 has negatively affected economic growth globally and if it continues for a long period could undermine Rwanda's path of export-led growth. The strong reliance on international assistance could weaken Rwanda's efforts at self-sustained growth. Food security is not guaranteed—the agricultural sector needs resources and inputs. A key question related to political development will occur in 2017 when President Kagame (if he wins his second term in 2010) will not be able to run for office again. Will Rwanda go the way of Uganda under its current President, Yoweri Museveni who successfully re-wrote the constitution to serve additional terms? The strength of the grassroots democratization and accountability programs, the political freedoms for the media, the gathering strength of new political leaders, parties and the Parliament, and the unique vision of President Kagame and his top leaders that is embedded in the constitution, make this path extremely unlikely.

One of the greatest challenges facing Rwanda is not internal but the world's continued ignorance and indifference which allows genocide deniers to re-write the history of the past and now deny the story of change and development to emerge. Most of the world, once again, is ignoring Rwanda.

On April 7, 2009, I sat with a delegation of scholars on a hill in Nyanza outside Kigali to commemorate the 15th commemoration of the genocide. It was the site where over 5,000 defenseless Tutsi's were massacred when UNAMIR troops first refused to use their weapons to protect those who were huddled in the schools, then withdrew, allowing the Interhamwe to do what they called "their work."

"We asked them to kill us rather than leave us to be hacked to death by machetes," said one of the very few survivors of the massacre who spoke at the commemoration ceremony.

Fifteen years ago, in 1994 on the beautiful hills of Rwanda, as thousands of innocent people were being brutally murdered, as corpses piled up in classrooms and churches, the world remained silent. It is hard for many in the West to believe that the French would play a role in supporting mass murders, but they did. It is hard for people to believe that the Catholic Church had a major role in the genocide as it built up over decades and that priests actually participated, but they did. It is hard for Americans to believe that the United States actively lobbied the United Nations Security Council to remove troops from Rwanda at the height of the killings, but they did. It is hard for people to believe that Human Rights Watch would ignore the truth but they are. It is hard to contemplate what happened in Rwanda fifteen years ago, but we owe it to all who perished to uncover the truth.

There are so many questions remaining: Why did the US choose not to intervene? Why did the French support the genocidal regime—with arms, training, French troops and with their power in the international community? Why have the French been allowed to indict President Kagame and members of his staff and Parliament who stopped the genocide while the world turned away, for "precipitating the genocide," without outrage from the international community? Why has the Catholic Church failed to act against the clergy (women and men) who have been convicted by the courts, those implicated in the genocide, and the many in hiding in Europe?

Why were many of the churches killing places instead of places of refuge?" Several times a day the priest would drag people out of the church and shoot them in the courtyard of Saint Famille Church," said Bonaventure. Why? The killers were certain the world would remain silent, and they were right.

Much of the world remains silent and indifferent now as those who supported the killers continue to shape the post-genocide debate. By being silent we are allowing the deniers and revisionists to shape the post genocide debate about Rwanda.

Gerald Caplan, a Canadian academic, has categorized the deniers and the revisionists into three categories. First are the genocidiares who have never been caught. They are not only in the Congo where they fled after the genocide but also in Belgium, France, Canada and the United States. Why are these killers allowed to life their lives free of impunity?

There are deniers and revisionists who seem to hate the RPF and Paul Kagame. These are people like the former hotel manager of the Mille Colline, made famous by the movie Hotel Rwanda, who now denies the genocide and says it was in invention of the RPF. Instead the world should hear from Jean de Dieu Mucyo, a lawyer who chaired the Commission on the Role of the French and now heads the National Commission for the Fight Against Genocide who was in the hotel. He tells his personal story of how his family and others—who were totally powerless—were told "give me money in exchange for your life."

There is another group who has made careers out of denying and denigrating the genocide who have built up a strong network that feeds off each other. Some of them are academics. One was on the campus of my university and said "there was no genocide."

Denial of what really happened denial of the progress that is occurring, is "like another cut with a machete,"[1] as Caplan said.

Those who are interested in the truth of what happened, those interested in understanding the unique experiment in reconciliation and hope that is occurring in Rwanda must continue to do honest research and scholarship based on evidence.

President Kagame who spoke eloquently at the end of the ceremony on April 7, 2009 in Nyanza said, "It is very difficult to build a country on human ashes," but then concluded with a Kinyarwanda saying: *Ukuri Guca Muziko Ntigushye* which means: truth goes through fire and is not burnt. We hope that this book contributes in some small way to the truth of post-genocide Rwanda.

At the end of the ceremony in Nyanza, a group of children approached the platform to sing. A very young girl, perhaps age five or six took the microphone and she said in a clear and strong voice:

"The world wonders whether we can rebuild after our terrible tragedy. Yes, we can," she said, "Yes we can."

Note

1. "Revisionism Well and Truly Alive," *The New Times*, April 7, 2009. P. 3.

Appendix

Primary Interviews: 1998-2009

Title of interviewee is based on their position when they were interviewed.

Bavugamenshi, Daniel. Chairman Association of Microfinance Institutions in Rwanda (AMIR)

Bayingana, Moses. National Coordinator: NICI Implementation Plan, Rwanda Information Technology Authority (RITA)

Bernadette, Honorable Kanzayire, Member of Parliament

Besage, Sarah, Headmistress, FAWE

Berry, John A. Microfinance Development Advisor, U.S. Agency for International Development (USAID)

Binagwaho, Dr. Agnes, Director of the National AIDS Committee

Butare, Albert. Vice-Rector, Kigali Institute of Science and Technology (KIST)

Carrell, Aileen. Manager: Green Coffee Sustainability Starbucks Coffee Company, Seattle, WA

Carter, Linda Professor, McGeorge School of Law, University of the Pacific, Sacramento, California

Chantal. Rosette. Director General, Rwanda Office of Tourism and National Parks

Fullerton, Peter. Director-General Rwanda Information Technology Authority (RITA)

Gallimore, Timothy. International Criminal Tribunal for Rwanda, Arusha, Tanzania

Ganza, Jean Baptiste. Jesuit School of Theology, University of California, Berkeley

Gasana, Javier. Assistant to the Minister of State for Primary and Secondary Education, Ministry of Education

Gatare, Francis Director-General Rwanda Investment and Export Promotion Agency

Hakizabera, Pipien. Director General. Centre for Support to Small and Medium-Sized Enterprise in Rwanda (CAPMER)

Hategeka, Emmanuel Secretary General Rwanda Private Sector Federation (RPSF)

Hoots, Cindy. Project Specialist: Corporate Social Responsibility, Starbucks Coffee Company, Seattle, Washington

Hughes, Mike Advisor: Research Science and Technology Office of the President

Inyumba, Aloysie, Member of Parliament, Republic of Rwanda

Johnson, Pamela. Executive Vice-President VOXIVA. Washington D.C.

Kabahizi, Celestin. Vice-Rector, Kigali Institute of Education

Kabuye, Rose Chief of Protocol, Office of the President, Republic of Rwanda

Kacyira, Dr. Aisa Kirabo. Mayor of Kigali, Rwanda

Kagame, President Paul. President of the Republic of Rwanda

Kaija, Barbara. Deputy Editor-in-Chief, *The New Vision*, Kampala, Uganda

Kali-Baingana, Maggie Lawyer and development expert

Kantarama, Penelope, Governor of the Western Province, Rwanda

Karas, Andy. Acting Mission Director USAID, Rwanda

Karega, Vincent. Minister of Commerce and Industry

Karugarama, Tharcisse

Karuretwa, Kaliza. Second Counsellor, Trade and Investment. Embassy of the Republic of Rwanda, Washington D.C.

Kimenyi, Alexandre. Professor of Linguistics, Ethnic studies and Pan-African Languages, California State University, Sacramento, California

Kimonyo, James. Ambassador to the United States of America

Lifa, Jonathan Francis Africa Regional Manager: Policy Government and Public Affairs. Chevron International Exploration and Production Company

Lwakambamba, Professor Silas. Rector: National University of Rwanda

Macrae, David. Ambassador, Head of Delegation. Delegation of the European Commission in Rwanda

Maniraguha, Alain Assistant, Minister of State in Charge of Industry and Investment Promotion

Manzi, Antoine Rutayisire. Director: Entrepreneurship Development and Business Growth, Private Sector Federation, Kigali, Rwanda

Mosupye, Dr. Boatamo Associate Professor of Ethnic Studies and Director of Pan African Studies, California State University, Sacramento, California

Mugambage, Major General Frank Director of Cabinet, Office of the President

Mukantabana, Mathilde. Professor of History, Consumes River College, Sacramento, California

Mukawamariya, Dr. Jeanne d'Arc. Secretary in Charge of Primary and Secondary, Ministry of Education, Republic of Rwanda

Mukantaganzwa, Domitilla. Executive Secretary: National Service of Gacaca Jurisdictions, Republic of Rwanda

Munyakazi, Dr. Louis. Director General National Institute of Statistics

Munyemana, Eric. Managing Director: Agape

Murego, John Vianney Gatsibo District Mayor

Murekeraho, Joseph. Secretary in Charge of Primary and Secondary, Ministry of Education, Republic of Rwanda

Mureramanzi, Professor Silas. Academic Vice-Rector, National University of Rwanda

Musoni, Protais. Minister of Local Governance, Community and Social Development, Republic of Rwanda

Mutanguha, Odette Coordinator: Forum for African Women Educationalists (FAWE) Rwanda Chapter

Murenzi, Romain: Minister of Education, Minister in Charge of Science and Technology

Murigande, Dr. Charles. Minister of Foreign Affairs and Cooperation, Republic of Rwanda

Mutanguha, Zephyr. Director: CAMERWA, Kigali, Rwanda

Ndahiro, Dr. Alfred. Adviser: Communication and Public Relations, Office of the President, Republic of Rwanda

Ndahiro, Tom, Former Human Rights Commissioner, Author

Ngarambe, Francois Xavier. Executive Secretary: Financial Sector Development Program. Ministry of Finance, Republic of Rwanda

Ngoga, Martin. Prosecutor General of the Republic, Republic of Rwanda

Niwemfura, Aquiline. Executive Secretary: Permanent Executive Secretariat for Beijing PFA Follow-Up

Nkusi, Professor Laurant. Minister of Information, Republic of Rwanda

Nsanzabaganwa, Monique: Secretary in Charge of Economic Plans, Ministry of Finance

Nsengimana, Professor Joseph. Ambassador: Permanent Representative Permanent Mission to the United Nations

Ntidendereza, William. Mayor: District of Kicukoro, City of Kigali

Nyabutsitsi, Gerard. Vice-Rector: Administration and Finance. Kigali Institute of Science and Technology (KIST)

Nyibizi, Bonaventure. President CogeBanque, Kigali, Rwanda

Nyiramilimo, Dr. Odette. Senator and Chairperson: Social Affairs, Human Rights and Petitions Committee

Ngoga, Mugunga, Remy. Economic Advisor, Office of the President, Republic of Rwanda

Nrirahabineza, Valerie. Minister in Charge of Family and Gender, Government of Rwanda Patrick, Henderson. Missions Director U.S. Agency for International Development (USAID)

Rugambwa, Alphonse. Coordinator: Protection and Care of Families against HIV/AIDS PACFA) Rwanda

Rusanga, Professor Martin. Club President: Rotary Club of Kigali Virunga

Taylor, Sandra Senior Vice-President Corporate Social Responsibility Starbucks Coffee Company, Seattle, Washington

Rwamasirabo, Emile. Rector, National University of Rwanda; Ambassador of the Republic of Rwanda to Japan

Schilling, Dr. Michelle Director: Geographic Information Systems and Remote Sensing Training and Research Centre. National University of Rwanda

Shyaka, Dr. Anastase. Director of CCM, National University of Rwanda, Butare, Rwanda

Uhiriwe, Mary. Project Officer: Protection and Care of Families against HIV/AIDS (PACFA) Rwanda

Umukobwa, Bellancille National President, AVEGA

Zirimwabagabo, Irene U. Communication Officer, United Nations Fund for Women (UNIFEM) Kigali, Rwanda

Zsenga, Dr. Zachary Ambassador to the United States of America and Secretary General Ministry of Defense

Bibliography

African Rights, *Rwanda: Death, Despair and Defiance*. London: African Rights, 1995.

African Peer Review for New Partnership for African Development (NEPAD). *Country Review of the Republic of Rwanda*, New Partnership for African Development , 2005.

Alkire, Sabina. "Why the Capability Approach?" *Journal of Human Development* Vol. 6. No 1. (2005): 115-133.

Arnold, Jobb. "Individual and Social Transformations: Growth and Reconciliation in Rwanda." Paper Presented at the First Interdiciplinary Conference on Genocide and Post-Genocide, Kigali Rwanda, July 2008.

Barnett, Michael. *Eyewitness to Genocide: The United Nations and Rwanda*. Ithaca: Cornell University Press, 2002.

Barro, Robert J. "Democracy and Growth." *Journal of Economic Growth* (March 1996): 1-27.

Batterbury, Simon and Jude Fernando. "Rescaling Governance and the Impacts of Political and Environmental Decentralization." *World Development* Vol. 34 No 11 (2006): 1851-1863.

Baum, Matthew. "Circling the Wagons: Soft News and Isolationism in American Public Opinion." Paper presented at the annual meeting of the American Political Science Association August 29-September 3, 2002.

Bertrand, William. "Progress and Challenges in Health Care and Information Technology in Rwanda." Paper presented at the Post-Genocide Rwanda Conference, California State University, Sacramento, CA. November 2-3, 2007.

Birdsall, Nancy. "Population Growth: Its Magnitude and Implications for Development." *Finance and Development* (1984): 10-15.

Brea, Jennifer. "The New Rwanda." *The Guardian*, 16 July 2007.

Brookings Institution: "Working Towards Universal Health Coverage in Rwanda." May 21, 2008.

Bulatao, R. *Reducing Fertility in Developing Countries: A Review of Determinants and Policy Levers*. Washington, D.C. The World Bank, 1984.

Busingye, Johnston. "Reality and Challenges of Legal and Judicial Reconstruction in Rwanda," Paper presented at the Legal and Judicial Reform in Post-Conflict Situations and the Role of the International Committee, The Hague Seminar December 7, 2006.

Carpio, Maria Abigail. "VUP Financial Services Component: Proposed Framework and Operating Guidelines." *Oxford Policy Management*, February 2009.

Chatterjee, Shiladitya. "Poverty Reduction Strategies-Lessons from the Asian and Pacific Region on Inclusive Development." *Asian Development Review* Vol. 22 No. 1 (2005): 12-44.

Cheema, G. Shabbir and Dennis Rondinelli, eds. *Decentralizing Governance: Emerging Concepts and Practices*. Washington, D.C.: Brookings Institution Press, 2007.

Clark, Phil and Zachary Kaufman eds. *After Genocide: Transitional Justice, Post-Conflict Reconstruction and Reconciliation in Rwanda and Beyond*. New York: Columbia University Press, 2009.

Clark, Phil. "The Rules (and Politics) of Engagement: The *Gacaca* Courts and Post-Genocide Justice, Healing and Reconciliation in Rwanda." In Phil Clark and Zachary Kaufman eds. *After Genocide: Transitional Justice, Post-Conflict Reconstruction and Reconciliation in Rwanda and Beyond*. New York: Columbia University Press, 2009.

Collier, Paul. *The Bottom Billion: Why the Poorest Countries are Failing and What Can be Done About It*. New York: Oxford University Press, 2007.

Crocker, David A. "Deliberative Participation in Local Development." *Journal of Human Development* Vol. 8 No. 3 (November, 2007): 431-55.

Dallaire, R. *Shake Hands with the Devil: The Failure of Humanity in Rwanda*. Toronto: Random House Canada, 2003.

Des Forges, A. *Leave None to Tell the Story: Genocide in Rwanda* New York: Human Rights Watch, 1999.

De Lorenzo, Mauro. "Rwanda Redux." *The American* (2006): 116-117.

Demographic and Health Survey: Rwanda. Calverton, Maryland: ORC Macro, 2006.

Destexhe, Alain. *Rwanda and Genocide in the Twentieth Century.* New York: New York University Press, 1995.

Devlin, Claire and Robert Elgie. "The Effect of Increased Women's Representation in Parliament: The Case of Rwanda." *Parliamentary Affairs* Vol. 61 Issue 2 (April, 2008): 237-254.

Diedhiou, Alpha. "Governance for Development: Understanding the Concept/Reality Linkages." *Journal of Human Development* Vol. 8 No. 1 (March, 2007): 23-38.

Doorknobs, Martin. "Good Governance: The Metamorphosis of a Policy Metaphor." *Journal of International Affairs* Vol. 57, No. 1 (2003): 3-17.

Drezner, Daniel. "Foreign Policy Goes Glam." *The National Interest* (November/December 2007): 22-28.

Drydrk, Jay. "When is Development More Democratic?" *Journal of Human Development* Vol. 6 No. 2 (July, 2005): 247-67.

Dougherty, Carter. "Rwanda Savors the Rewards of Coffee Production." New York Times, November 3, 2006, 1-3.

Easterly, William. "How the Millennium Development Goals are Unfair to Africa." Brookings Institution Global Economy and Development Working Paper 14. (November 2007): 1-23.

Easterly, William. "Planners Versus Searchers in Foreign Aid." *Asian Development Review* Vol. 23, No. 1 (2006): 1-35.

Easterly, William. *The Elusive Quest for Growth: Economists' Adventures and Misadventures in the Tropics.* Cambridge: MIT Press, 2002.

Ensign, Margee. "Learning from Rwanda" OP-ED *The Record*, July, 2007.

Ensign, Margee. "Political, Economic and Social Progress in Rwanda Thirteen Years after the Genocide." Paper presented at the Post-Genocide Rwanda Conference, California State University, Sacramento, CA. November 2-3, 2007.

Ensign, Margee. "Imihigo and Local Governance in Rwanda." Presented at the Urban Institute, Washington D.C., April, 2007.

Ensign, Margee. "History and Hope: Progress in Rwanda." Paper presented at the First Annual Interdisciplinary Conference on Genocide and Post-Genocide. Kigali, Rwanda July 2008.

Ensign, Margee. "What We Don't Know About the World." *San Francisco Chronicle*, Op-Ed, April 11, 2005.

Evans, Peter. "Collective Capabilities, Culture and Amartya Sen's Development as Freedom." Studies in Comparative International Development Vol. 37, No. 2 (Summer 2002): 54-60.

Evans, A, Piron, L, Curran, Z. and Driscoll, R. *Independent Evaluation of Rwanda's Poverty Reduction Strategy 2002-2005*, Final Report ODI/IDS, 2005.

"Fast Cities, 2008." *Fast Company* (June 2008): 85-86.

FAWE Rwanda Celebrates its 10th Anniversary, FAWE Rwanda Newsletter, December 2006.

FAWE Rwanda "Speak Out Process," 2005.

FAWE Rwanda Newsletter (January-April, 2007).

Fowler, Jerry. "The Church and Power: Responses to Genocide and Massive Human Rights Abuses in Comparative Perspective." In Rittner, Carol John K. Roth and Wendy Whitworth. *Genocide in Rwanda: Complicity of the Churches?* Newark, U.K.: Aegis Publishers, 2004.

Fritz, Verena and Alina Rocha Menocal. "Developmental States in the New Millennium: Concepts and Challenges for a New Aid Agenda." *Development Policy Review* Vol. 25, No. 5 (2007): 531-552.

Gallimore, Timothy. "The Legacy of the International Criminal Tribunal for Rwanda (ICTR) and its Contributions to Justice and Reconciliation in Rwanda." Paper presented at the Post-Genocide Rwanda Conference, California State University, Sacramento, CA. November 2-3, 2007.

Goulet, Denis. "Participation in Development: New Avenues." *World Development* Vol. 17 No. 2 (1989): 165-78.

Government of Rwanda, Ministry of Education, Science, Technology and Scientific Research. Education Sector Strategic Plan: 2004-08.

Government of Rwanda Vision 2020 Umurenge: An Integrated Local Development Program to Accelerate Poverty Eradication, Rural Growth and Social Protection." EDPRS Flagship Program Document, August, 2007.

Grindle, Merilee. "Good Enough Governance Revisited." *Development Policy Review* Vol. 25 No. 5 (2007): 553-574.

Grindle, Merilee S. *Going Local: Decentralization, Democratization and the Promise of Good Governance* Princeton: Princeton University Press, 2007.

Gourevitch, Philip. *We Wish to Inform You that Tomorrow We Will be Killed With Our Families: Stories from Rwanda.* New York: Farrar, Straus and Giroux, 1998.

Haddad, Wadi. *Education and Development: Evidence for New Priorities.* Washington, D.C.: The World Bank, 1990.

Hamoudi, Amar and Jeffrey D. Sachs. "Economic Consequences of Health Status: A Review of the Evidence." Harvard University Center for International Development Working Paper No. 30 (December 1999) 1-25.

Hatry, Harry. "Emerging Developments in Performance Measurement: An International Perspective." In Julnes, Patria de Lancer, Frances Stokes Berry, Maria Aristigueta, and Kaifeng Yang eds. *International Handbook of Practice-Based Performance Management.* London: Sage, 2008.

Hayman, Rachel. "Are the MDGs Enough? Donor Perspectives and Recipient Visions of Education and Poverty Reduction in Rwanda." *International Journal of Educational Development* Vol. 27 (2007): 371-382.

Holzer, Marc and Kathryn Kloby. "Helping Government Measure Up: Models of Citizen Driven Government Performance Measurement Initiatives." Julnes, Patria de Lancer, Frances Stokes Berry, Maria Aristigueta, and Kaifeng Yang eds. *International Handbook of Practice-Based Performance Management.* London: Sage, 2008.

Huggins, Allison and Shirley Randell. "Gender Equality in Education in Rwanda: What is Happening to our Girls?" Paper presented at the South African Association of Women Graduates Conference on "Dropouts from School and Tertiary Studies," Capetown, South Africa May, 2007.

Hjelle, Benjamin. "From Arusha to the Hague: Constructing International Criminal Justice Regimes." Paper presented at the Post-Genocide Rwanda Conference, California State University, Sacramento, CA. November 2-3, 2007.

Hochschild, Adam. *King Leopold's Ghost: A Story of Greed, Terror and Heroism in Colonial Africa.* New York: Houghton Mifflin, 1998.

Hunter-Gault, Charlayne. *New News Out of Africa: Uncovering Africa's Renaissance.* New York: Oxford University Press, 2006.

International Labor Organization. *Employment Growth and Basic Needs: A One World Problem.* Geneva: ILO, 1976.

"Imidugu Elections" *Africa Research Bulletin.* August, 2006.

International Monetary Fund. *Rwanda: Joint Staff Assessment of the Poverty Reduction Strategy Paper: Progress Report.* IMF Country Report No. 04/274. August, 2004.

International Monetary Fund and International Development Association. *Joint Staff Advisory Note of the Poverty Reduction Strategy Paper: Annual Progress Report.* March 22, 2005.

International Monetary Fund and International Development Association. *Joint Staff Advisory Note of the Poverty Reduction Strategy Paper: Annual Progress Report.* March 27, 2006.

International Monetary Fund. *Final Evaluation Report of Rwanda's Poverty Reduction Strategy (2002),* July, 2006.

Izabiliza, Jeanne. "The Role of Women in Reconstruction: Experience of Rwanda." Unpublished paper.

International Research and Exchange Board, (IREX), Media Sustainability Index for Africa 2006-2007 www.irex.org/programs/MSI_Africa/rwanda.asp.

Johns Hopkins Center for Communications Programs. *Perceptions about the Gacaca Law in Rwanda: Evidence from a Multi-Method Study.* Special Publication No. 19. Baltimore: Johns Hopkins University School of Public Health, Center for Communication Programs. April, 2001.

Jolly, Richard. L. Emmerij and Thomas Weiss. "The Power of UN Ideas: Lessons from the first 60 Years." *The United Nations Intellectual History Project.* London: Grundy and Northedge, 2005.

Julnes, Patria de Lancer, Frances Stokes Berry, Maria Aristigueta, and Kaifeng Yang eds. *International Handbook of Practice-Based Performance Management.* London: Sage, 2008.

Kakwani, Nanak and Ernesto Pernia. "What is Pro-Poor Growth?" *Asian Development Review* Vol. 18, No. 1 (2000): 1-16.

Kaplinsky, Raphel and Dirk Messner. "Introduction: The Impact of Asian Drivers on the Developing World." *World Development* Vol. 36, No. 2 (2007): 197-209.

Kaufmann, D., A. Kraay and M. Mastruzzi. *Governance Matters VII: Governance Indicators for 1996-2007.* Washington D.C.: The World Bank, 2008.

Kroslak, Daniela. *The French Betrayal of Rwanda.* Bloomington: Indiana University Press, 2008.

Landesman, Peter. "The Minister of Rape." *New York Times Magazine,* September 15, 2002, 82-89.

Manor, James. "Democratisation with Inclusion: Political Reforms and People's Empowerment at the Grassroots." *Journal of Human Development* Vol. 5, No. 1 (March, 2004): 5-29.

Macmillan Rwanda: *Primary Social Studies Pupil's Book 5*. Macmillan Rwanda, 2006.

Macmillan Rwanda: *Primary Social Studies Pupil's Book 6*. Macmillan Rwanda, 2006.

McNeill, Desmond. "Human Development: The Power of the Idea." *Journal of Human Development* Vol. 8, No. 1 (March 2007): 5-22.

Melvern, Linda. *Conspiracy to Murder: The Rwandan Genocide*. London: Versco, 2004.

Melvern, L.R. *A People Betrayed: The Role of the West in Rwanda's Genocide*. London: Zed Books, 2000.

Melvern, Linda. "The Past is Prologue: Planning the 1994 Genocide." In Clark, Phil and Zachary Kaufman eds. *After Genocide: Transitional Justice, Post-Conflict Reconstruction and Reconciliation in Rwanda and Beyond*. New York: Columbia University Press, 2009.

Ministere De L'Administration Locale et des Affaires Sociales, Programme National de Renforcement de la Bonne Gouvernance our la Reduction de la Pauvrete au Rwanda. Kigali, Rwanda, Mai, 2002.

Misuraca, Gianluca. *E-Governance in Africa: From Theory to Action*. Trenton, N.J.: Africa World Press, 2007.

Mladovsky, Philipa and Elias Mossialos. "A Conceptual Framework for Community-Based Health Insurance in Low-Income Countries: Social Capital and Economic Development." *World Development* Vol. 36, No. 4 (2008): 590-607.

Munyaneza, James. "Kagame Wins 2007 Africa Gender Award." AllAfrica.com January 28, 2007.

Murenzi, Professor Romain. "Africa in the Global Knowledge Economy." *In Going for Growth: Science, Technology and Innovation in Africa, edited by Professor Calestous Juma, 48-61. London: The Smith Institute, 2005.*

Mutume, Gumisai. "Women Break Into African Politics." *Africa Recovery* Vol. 18, No. 1 (April 2004): 1-6.

Narayan, Deepa ed. *Measuring Empowerment: Cross-Disciplinary Perspectives*. Washington, D.C.: The World Bank, 2000.

Ndahiro, Tom. "The Church's Blind Eye to Genocide in Rwanda." In Rittner, Carol John K. Roth and Wendy Whitworth *Genocide in*

Rwanda: Complicity of the Churches? Newark, U.K.: Aegis Publishers, 2004.

Ndahiro, Tom. "Genocide-Laundering: Historical Revisionism, Genocide Denial and the Rassemblement Republicain our la Democratie au Rwanda." In Clark, Phil and Zachary Kaufman eds. *After Genocide: Transitional Justice, Post-Conflict Reconstruction and Reconciliation in Rwanda and Beyond.* New York: Columbia University Press, 2009.

Ndulu, Benno. *Challenges of African Growth: Opportunities, Constraints and Strategic Directions.* Washington, D.C.: The World Bank, 2007.

New York Times, "Coffee and Hope Grow in Rwanda." April 6, 2006.

Nyangara, Florence, Camilee Hart, Ilene Speizer and Scott Moreland. *Unmet Need for Family Planning in Rwanda and Madagascar: An Analysis Report for the Repositioning of Family Planning Initiatives.* Chapel Hill, Carolina Population Center, University of North Carolina, April, 2007.

Ngoga, Martin. "The Institutionalism of Impunity: A Judicial Perspective of the Rwandan Genocide," In Phil Clark and Zachary Kaufman eds. *After Genocide: Transitional Justice, Post-Conflict Reconstruction and Reconciliation in Rwanda and Beyond.* New York: Columbia University Press, 2009.

Olowu, Dele and James Wunsch. *Local Governance in Africa: The Challenges of Democratic Decentralization.* Boulder: Lynne Reinner Publishers, 2004.

O'Neill, William S.J. "Hoping Against Hope: The Ethics of Social Reconciliation." Paper presented at the First Annual Interdisciplinary Conference on Genocide and Post-Genocide. Kigali, Rwanda July, 2008.

Organization for Social Science Research in Eastern and Southern Africa. (OSSRESA) *Rwanda: Citizen Report Cards and Community Score Cards.* OSSRESA, 2006.

Oxhorn, Philip, Joseph S. Tulchin and Andrew D. Selee. *Decentralization, Democratic Governance and Civil Society in Comparative Perspective: Africa, Asia and Latin America.* Baltimore: Johns Hopkins University Press, 2004.

PEPFAR (President's Emergency Plan for AIDS Relief): Rwanda TRACnet enhances monitoring of ART Scale Up" www.pepfar.gov February, 2006.

Peterson, Scott. *Me Against My Brother: At War in Somalia, Sudan and Rwanda*. New York: Routledge, 2000.

Power, Samantha. "Rwanda: The Two Faces of Justice." *The New York Review* (January 16, 2003) 47-50.

Power, Samantha. *"A Problem from Hell": America and the Age of Genocide*. New York: Harper Collins, 2003.

Power, Samantha. "Bystanders to Genocide." *The Atlantic* (September 2001). Vol. 288. No. 2.

Powley, Elizabeth. "Rwanda: The Impact of Women Legislators on Policy Outcomes Affecting Children and Families." Background Paper: The State of the World's Children, UNICEF, 2007.

Prunier, Gerard. *The Rwanda Crisis: History of Genocide*. New York: Columbia University Press, 1995.

Randall, Vicky. "Political Parties and Democratic Developmental States." *Development Policy Review* Vol. 25, No. 5 (2007): 633-652.

Ranis, Gustav, Francis Stewart and Emma Samman. "Human Development: Beyond the Human Development Index." *Journal of Human Development* Vol. 7. No. 3 (November 2006): 323-357.

Ravallion, Martin. "Are There Lessons for Africa from China's Success Against Poverty?" World Bank Policy Research Working Paper No. 4463, Washington D.C., The World Bank, January 2008.

Republic of Rwanda, Economic Development and Poverty Reduction Strategy 2008-2012.

Republic of Rwanda, Ministry of Finance and Economic Planning. Rwanda Vision 2020, 2000.

Republic of Rwanda, Ministry of Finance and Economic Planning, Poverty Reduction Strategy. Policy Matrix, July, 2005.

Republic of Rwanda, Ministry of Finance and Economic Planning. Annual Economic Reports, 2005-07.

Republic of Rwanda, Ministry of Finance and Economic Planning. National Microfinance Policy, September, 2006.

Republic of Rwanda, Ministry of Finance and Economic Planning. (2007) EDPRS Poverty Analysis of Ubudehe, Republic of Rwanda, Kigali.

Republic of Rwanda, Ministry of Health. Health Sector Policy February, 2005.

Republic of Rwanda, Ministry of Health. Mutual Health Insurance Policy in Rwanda December, 004.

Republic of Rwanda, Ministry of Health. The Center for the Treatment and Research on HIV/AIDS and Malaria, Tuberculosis and other epidemics. www.moh.gov.rw/docs/trac+presentation.pdf.

Republic of Rwanda, Ministry of Health. National Health Accounts, Rwanda 2006: HIV/AIDS, Malaria and Reproductive Health.

Republic of Rwanda, Ministry of Local Government and Social Affairs. Community Development Policy, May, 2000.

Republic of Rwanda, Ministry of Local Government and Social Affairs. Plan de Developpement du District de Gatsibo, 2008-20012.

Republic of Rwanda, Ministry of Local Government and Social Affairs. Making Decentralised Service Delivery Work: Putting the People at the centre of Service Provision, Policy Note, Kigali, 2006.

Republic of Rwanda, Ministry of Local Government and Social Affairs. The Matrix of Roles and Responsibilities for Decentralized Service Delivery Annex 1, 2006.

Republic of Rwanda, Ministry of Local Government and Social Affairs. National Decentralization Policy. May, 2000.

Republic of Rwanda, Ministry of Local Government and Social Affairs. Implementation Strategy for National Decentralization Policy. May, 2000.

Republic of Rwanda, Ministry of Local Governance. (2006) Making Decentralised Service Delivery Work: Putting the People at the centre of Service Provision, Policy Note, Kigali.

Republic of Rwanda, Ministry of Local Government and Social Affairs. National Decentralization Policy. May, 2000.

Republic of Rwanda, Ministry of Local Government and Social Affairs. Implementation Strategy for National Decentralization Policy. May, 2000.

Republic of Rwanda, National Service of Gacaca Courts, Summary, 2006.

Republic of Rwanda, National Service of Gacaca Courts: Process of Collecting Information Requited in Gacaca Courts, November 2004.

Republic of Rwanda, National Service of Gacaca Courts: Trial Procedure in Gacaca Courts, January, 2005.

Republic of Rwanda, 2003 Constitution.

Republic of Rwanda, Organic Education Law.

Republic of Rwanda, Ministry of Local Government, Good Governance, Community Development and Social Affairs. Rwanda's Decentralized Governance Reform Policy August, 2005.

Republic of Rwanda, Rwanda Investment and Export Promotion Agency (REIPA): Annual Reports 2005-06.

Rettig, Max. "Gacaca: Results from a Multimodal Study." Paper presented at the Post-Genocide Rwanda Conference, California State University, Sacramento, CA. November 2-3, 2007.

Rittner, Carol John K. Roth and Wendy Whitworth. *Genocide in Rwanda: Complicity of the Churches?* Newark, U.K.: Aegis Publishers, 2004.

Robeyns, Ingrid. "The Capability Approach: A Theoretical Survey." *Journal of Human Development* Vol. 6 No. 1 (March 2005): 94-114.

Rodrik, Dani. "Development Lessons for Asia from Non-Asian Countries." *Asian Development Review* Vol. 23, No. 1 (2006): 1-15.

Rodrick, Dani, ed. *In Search of Prosperity: Analytic Narratives on Economic Growth.* Princeton: Princeton University Press, 2003.

Rodrick, Dani. "Rethinking Growth Strategies," in A.B. Atkinson et al., WIDER Perspectives on Global Development, Palgrave-Macmillan in association with UNU-WIDER, London, 2005.

The Luca d'Agliano Lecture in Development Economics Delivered October 8, 2004.

Roy, Indrajit. "Civil Society and Good Governance: (Re-) Conceptualizing the Interface. *World Development* Vol. 36, No. 4 (2008): 677-705.

Rusagara, Frank. "Gacaca: Rwanda's Truth and Reconciliation Authority." Paper presented at the First Annual Interdisciplinary Conference on Genocide and Post-Genocide. Kigali, Rwanda July 2008.

Rwanda National Examinations Council. "The Structure of the Education System in Rwanda and the System of Evaluation in Secondary Schools."

"Rwanda: Pension Bodies Laud Country's Health Insurance." allAfrica.com 19, November 2008.

Sachs, Jeffrey ed. *Developing Country Debt and Economic Performance.* Chicago: University of Chicago Press, 1989.

Saith, Ashwani. "From Universal Values to Development Goals: Lost in Translation." *Development and Change* Vol. 37, No. 6 (2006): 1167-1199.

Schabas, William A. "Post Genocide Justice in Rwanda: A Spectrum of Options." In Phil Clark and Zachary Kaufman eds. *After Genocide: Transitional Justice, Post-Conflict Reconstruction and Reconciliation in Rwanda and Beyond.* New York: Columbia University Press, 2009.

Scherrer, Christian P. *Genocide and Crisis in Central Africa: Conflict Roots, Mass Violence and Regional War.* Westport: Praeger Publishers, 2002.

Sen, Amartya. "Development Thinking at the Beginning of the 21st Century." Paper Presented at the Conference on Development Thinking and Practice, Inter-American Development Bank, Washington D.C. 3-5 September, 1996.

Sen, Amaryta. *Development as Freedom.* New York: Anchor Books, 2000.

Shah, Anwar ed. Measuring Government Performance in the Delivery of Public Services Washington, D.C.: The World Bank, 2003.

Shah, Anwar and Theresa Thompson. "Implementing Decentralized Local Governance: A Treacherous Road with Potholes, Detours and Road Closures." World Bank Policy Research Paper 3353, June 2004.

Shalita, Willis. "The Fallacy of the Movie Hotel Rwanda." Paper presented at the Post-Genocide Rwanda Conference, California State University, Sacramento, CA. November 2-3, 2007.

Shyaka, Anastase. "Genocide, Identity Questions, Government and Democracy in Rwanda," Paper presented at the Post-Genocide Rwanda Conference, California State University, Sacramento, CA. November 2-3, 2007.

Sirleaf, Ellen Johnson and Steven Radelet. "The Good News out of Africa: Democracy, Stability and the Renewal of Growth and Development," in *Visions of Growth: Global Perspectives for Tomorrow's Wellbeing* edited by Beatrice Weder di Mauro Berlin: Campus Verlag, 2008.

Smith, Zeric Kay, Timothy Longman, Jean Kimonyo and Theooneste Rutagengwa. "Rwanda Democracy and Governance Assessment: Final Report." USAID, November 2002.

Soeters, Robert, Christian Habineza and Peter Bob Peerenboom. "Performance-Based Financing and Changing the District Health System: Experience from Rwanda." *Bulletin of the World Health Organization* Vol. 84 No. 11 (November, 2006): 884-89.

Soeters, Robert and L. Musabgo. "Comparison of Two Output Schemes in Butare and Cyangugu Provinces with two Control Provinces in Rwanda," 2005 World Bank: *Global Partnership on Output-Based Aid* (GPOBA).

Stiglitz, Joseph E. ed. *Rethinking the East Asian Miracle.* New York: Oxford University Press, 2001.

Srinivasan, Sharath. "No Democracy without Justice: Amaryta Sen's unfinished business with the capability approach." Doctoral research, University of Oxford.

Streeten, Paul. *First Things First: Meeting Basic Human Needs in the Developing Countries*. New York: Oxford University Press, 1981.

Tamale, Sylvia. *When Hens Begin to Crow: Gender and Parliamentary Politics in Uganda*. Boulder: Westview Press, 1999.

Temple-Raston, Dina. Justice on the Grass: *Three Rwandan Journalists, their Trial for War Crimes, and a Nation's Quest for Redemption*. New York: Free Press, 2005.

Teschner, Douglass. "Analysis of the Legislative Process at the Rwanda Transitional National Assembly." USAID/ ARD/SUNY: Project d' Appui a L'Assemblee Nationale du Rwanda, September 19, 2002.

The Independent. "Rwanda: Road to Prosperity." August 1-7, 2008.

Thompson, Allan, ed. *The Media and the Rwanda Genocide*. London: Pluto Press, 2007.

Traylor, Adrian. "Why we Failed: An Interest Based Analysis of the Negotiation Before and During the 1994 Rwandan Genocide." Paper presented at the Post-Genocide Rwanda Conference, California State University, Sacramento, CA. November 2-3, 2007.

Treisman, Daniel. *The Architecture of Government: Rethinking Political Decentralization*. Cambridge: Cambridge University Press, 2007.

UNCTAD (2006). *Investment Policy Review Rwanda*, New York and Geneva.

UNDP (2007). *Rwanda: Human Development Report 2007*, New York, UNDP.

United Nations Department of Economic and Social Affairs (UNDESA) Promoting citizen Engagement in Public Revenue Generation: Rwanda Case Study, 2008.

United Nations Economic Commission for Africa: African Centre for Statistics: "Special Focus Africa in Global Statistical System." Volume 2 Issue 1 (March 2008) 1-52.

United Nations. *Report of the World Commission on Environment and Development: Our Common Future*. Document A/42/427 New York: The United Nations, 1987.

United Nations Resolution 999 S/RES/955 (8 November 1994).

USAID. *Politique Nationale de Sante de la Reproduction*, Kigali, July 2003.

USAID. "USAID and Rwandan Ambassador Celebrate Rwanda Coffee." Press Release, April 11, 2006.

USAID. *Rwanda Country Health Statistical Report*, May, 2007.

USAID. "Twubakane Decentralization and Health Program Rwanda Report #12" October-December 2007.

USAID. "Land Dispute Management in Rwanda: Final Report" June, 2008.

USAID. "Restoring Hope through Economic Opportunity: Final Report of the Agribusiness Development Assistance to Rwanda (ADAR) Project." 2007.

"Vansina, Jan. *Antecedents to Modern Rwanda: The Nyiginya Kingdom*. Madison: University of Wisconsin Press, 2004.

Vitro, Robert ed. The Knowledge Economy in Development: Perspectives for Effective Partnerships. Washington, D.C.: Inter-American Development Bank, 2005.

Wagner, Scott. "Progress and Challenges in Post-Genocide Rwanda." Paper presented at the Post-Genocide Rwanda Conference, California State University, Sacramento, CA. November 2-3, 2007.

Wingfield-Digby, Peter. "Africa's STATS League: The Movers and Shakers 2006-07." *African Statistical Newsletter* Vol. 2 Issue 1 (March, 2008): 26-33.

Winrock International Institute for Agricultural Development. *African Development: Lessons from Asia*. Washington D.C.: The Winrock Institute, 1991.

World Bank. *Education in Rwanda: Rebalancing Resources to Accelerate Post-Conflict Development and Poverty Reduction*. Washington, D.C.: The World Bank, 2004.

World Bank. *Engendering Development through Gender Equality in Rights, Resources and Voice*. Washington, D.C. The World Bank, 2001.

World Bank. *The East Asian Miracle: Economic Growth and Public Policy*. Washington, D.C. New York: Oxford University Press, 1993.

World Bank. *Rwanda Joint Governance Assessment Report*. World Bank Country Manager, Kigali Rwanda. August 3, 2008.

World Bank. *Toward a Conflict-Sensitive Poverty Reduction Strategy: Lessons from a Retrospective Analysis*. Report 32587, June 30, 2005. Washington, D.C.: The World Bank, 2005.

World Bank. *Agricultural Policy Note: Promoting Pro-Poor Growth in Rwanda: Challenges and Opportunities*, Washington D.C. The World Bank, 2006.

World Bank. *World Development Report, 2000/2001: Attacking Poverty*. Washington, D.C. World Bank, 2001.

World Bank. *World Development Report, 1993: Investing in Health*. Washington, D.C. World Bank, 1993.

World Bank. *Rwanda Country Economic Memorandum*, Washington D.C. The World Bank, 2007.

World Bank. "Doing Business: Rwanda in Top 20 Reformers Globally," December 3, 2008. http://www.worldbank.org/WBSITE/EXTERNAL/COUNTRIES.

"World Bank Sees Africa Progress." BBC News, August 7, 2007.

World Bank. *World Development Report 2008: Agriculture for Development*. Washington, D.C.: The World Bank, 2008.

Index

About the Authors

Margee M. Ensign is the Dean of the School of International Studies (SIS), and Associate Provost for International Initiatives at the University of the Pacific that has campuses in San Francisco (Dugoni School of Dentistry), Sacramento, (McGeorge School of Law) and the main campus located in Stockton. The School of International Studies offers both undergraduate and graduate degrees in international and intercultural relations and is establishing programs in social entrepreneurship and Inter-American affairs. It is the only undergraduate program in the U.S. that requires all students to study abroad for at least a semester.

Dr. Ensign came to Pacific from Washington, D.C., where she helped to establish a program for Tulane University focused on the study of international development which is now offered on four continents. She began her career at Columbia University's School of International and Public Affairs. Her academic publications have focused on international development, foreign assistance, and formal modeling using artificial intelligence. For the past decade she has worked on development projects in Central, East and West Africa, including a PEPFAR project in Rwanda.

William E. Bertrand currently holds the endowed Wisner Professorship at Tulane University and is active in teaching and research programs focused on health, technology, and development issues. Dr. Bertrand made his first trip to Central Africa in 1979 where he was the founder of the then Zaire National Nutrition Planning Center. He was an early proponent of the use of information technology in Africa, developing the first computerized national health information system in Niger (1983) followed by the development of and implementation of the Famine Early Warning System (FEWS) which still serves a the primary tool in the regions protection against famine. In 1986 he moved to Kinshasa where he was one of the founding Directors of the Kinshasa School of

Public Health. As a principle consultant to the Rockefeller Foundation Schools of Public Health Without Walls Initiative he helped to start African Schools of Public Health in Uganda, Zimbabwe, South Africa, Ghana, Senegal, and Rwanda. He directed Tulane University's programs in support of the PEPFAR HIV/AIDS initiative in Rwanda starting in 2002 and is currently serving as Director of the Payson Center project verifying the chocolate industries efforts to eliminate the worst forms of child labor in Ghana and the Ivory Coast.

At Tulane he has served as Chair of Biostatistics and Epidemiology; was the Founding Chair of the Department of International Health and the Founding Director of the Payson Center of International Development and Technology Transfer. The author of numerous articles on international development, Dr. Bertrand has also served on the National Institutes of Health (NIH) Council and the Board of the Pan American Health and Development Foundation. He is currently working with UNAIDS in expanding their work in impact evaluation.